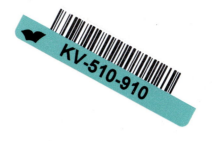

Rick Rogers is Education Correspondent for the *New Statesman*, and a freelance journalist and editor. He is a regular contributor to the *Guardian*, the *Times Educational Supplement*, and *Where*. Since studying English at Sussex University (1965-8), he has worked for Political and Economic Planning (1972-3), the Advisory Centre for Education as editor of *Where* (1974-7), the National Association of Citizens' Advice Bureaux, and the Association of Community Health Councils for England and Wales. He is the author of *Schools Under Threat: a Handbook on Closures* (1979), *Crowther to Warnock: How Fourteen Reports Tried to Change Children's Lives* (1980), and the editor of *Television and the Family* (1980). He is on the management committee of the national Children's Legal Centre, and a member of the advisory committee for CLEAR—the Campaign for Lead-free Air.

LEAD POISON

Rick Rogers

NS Report 7

©*Rick Rogers*

Typeset and designed by
Review Design Services
59 Whitworth St, Manchester 1

Printed by
Manchester Free Press
59 Whitworth St, Manchester 1
061-228 0976

Published by
New Statesman, 10, Great Turnstile, London WC1

ISBN 0 900962 12 7

Trade distribution by
Scottish & Northern Book Distributors Ltd,
18 Granby Row, Manchester 1

&

48A Hamilton Place, Edinburgh EH3 5AX

Southern Distribution
Albion Yard, 17A Balfe Street, London N1

Cover photograph—*Kevin Cummins*

Contents

Box information— What we use lead for; Lead workers;
Associated Octel; Other sources of lead
pollution; Lead study defects; graphs.

"Some of them gets lead-pisoned soon, and some of them gets lead-pisoned later, and some, but not many, niver; and 'tis all according to the constitooshun, sur; and some constitooshuns is strong and some is weak."

From "The Uncommercial Traveller"
by Charles Dickens, 1868.

LEAD pollution in Britain's cities is a serious environmental issue. It has also become a major educational one. For a substantial—some scientists now say overwhelming—body of high-quality evidence is showing that lead is having a devastating effect on children. Many develop disturbing behaviour problems or suffer impaired intellectual performance.

In short, we are poisoning our children—and the number could be as high as 95 per cent of all city-based children.

The chief cause of that pollution is leaded petrol. Other frequent, but more localised, sources include leaded paint, lead plumbing, certain cosmetics, glazed earthenware, industrial processes that use lead (such as smelters or battery firms), and used car dumps.

For several years controversy has raged among scientists and doctors over the seriousness of the danger that lead pollution poses for children. In spite of vigorous action by numerous industrialised countries to get rid of lead, successive British governments have accepted (and sometimes solicited) the views of those who claim there is no cause for concern. Ministers and civil servants have continued to set the wellbeing of children below the enhancement of commercial interests—notably the oil, lead and motor industries. Scientists and doctors who play down the lead danger have been found to have financial connections with those industries.

Gradually, official behaviour over lead pollution has changed from bland complacency to engineering a combination of depressing cover-ups and unsatisfactory compromises. In May 1981, the Government announced a reduction in the level of lead in petrol to be effective from the end of 1985. What this amounts to is that, having acknowledged the danger that lead poses, the government declined to act to eliminate that danger.

What then is the evidence against lead—and in particular against lead in petrol? How does lead affect us and our children? Where have the cover-ups been? What can we do to combat lead pollution?

Measuring lead

THREE KEY measurements recur throughout this publication.

ug/100ml
This relates to blood lead levels in humans. For example, 35ug/100ml means 35 micrograms of lead to a hundred millilitres of blood.

g/l
This relates to the lead content in petrol. For example, 0.40g/l means 0.40 grams of lead per litre of petrol.

ppm
This relates to the lead content in dust. For example, 500ppm means 500 parts of lead to a million parts of dust.

Lead in city schools

IN THE SUMMER of 1979, 28 inner London primary schools were tested at random for lead pollution. Twenty-five of those schools breached the safety level of lead in dust recommended by the US Environmental Protection Agency. Four schools were so polluted by lead and other metals they were causing Inner London Education Authority officials 'extreme concern'.

Yet both ILEA and the GLC, which carried out the survey refused to make public the names of the polluted schools 'in case parents panic or go wild'. Reports of the survey were sent to councillors on GLC and ILEA committees with the names of the schools omitted. Only one copy of the survey matching the names of the schools to the lead pollution readings existed in GLC files. The councillors accepted the need for secrecy and did not ask for the schools to be named. It was suggested that a further series of tests be carried out.

In April 1981, the *New Statesman* located the 28 schools involved and published a report of the suppressed survey.

The recommended 'safety level' for the amount of lead in dust is 500 parts of lead to a million parts of dust—500ppm. Even this is 30 times the natural level in an unpolluted soil-derived dust, 500 times the statutory maximum level in most food, and 2,500 times the maximum permitted level in food for babies. Three of the ILEA primary schools registered a dangerously high pollution level: Telferscot in Balham (5,190ppm), Rushmore in Clapton (4,730ppm) and Harbinger in Millwall (3,150ppm). The readings at these schools ranged from 120 up to a staggering 26,500ppm at Telferscot.

A fourth primary school—St Bernadette's, just round the corner from Telferscot—recorded an 'exceptionally high' arsenic and chromium pollution level. (Arsenic is commonly emitted from lead/zinc and copper smelters, and from some wood-preserving processes.) It was fifty times higher than the mean level for all playgrounds in London. No statutory levels for arsenic exist for the general environment, only for works atmospheres. But for land reclaimed from industrial dereliction for housing, the following guidelines apply for arsenic in soil: gardens 10 to 20ppm, amenity and open public spaces 40ppm. For American urban roadways the average reading is 11ppm. At St Bernadette's the arsenic level in the playground dust was 400ppm.

Two of the other 24 lead-risk schools (Phoenix and Beechcroft) cater for delicate or maladjusted children.

The full list of schools, with their lead readings, is:

School	Concentration of lead in playground dust (ppm)	
	mean	range
Telferscot, Telferscot Rd, SW12	5190	120-26500
Rushmore, Rushmore Rd, E5	4730	500-15700
Harbinger, Cahir St, E14	3150	1290- 4250
Henry Compton, Kingwood Rd, SW6	1990	830- 6950
Pakeman, Hornsey Rd, N7	1840	390- 3780
Bentworth, Bentworth Rd, W12	1800	660- 4110
St Thomas More, Appleton Rd, SE9	1350	320- 3550
Redriff, Rotherhithe St, SE16	1100	440- 3510
Penton, Ritchie St, N1	1010	260- 2130
Dulwich Village, Dulwich SE21	940	240- 3490
Seven Mills, Malabar St, E14	890	230- 2270
St Stephen's, Westbourne Park Rd, W2	890	420- 2460
Latchmere, Burns Rd, SW11	880	430- 1470
Drayton Park, N5	880	340- 1860
Phoenix, Bow Rd, E3	880	170- 2990
Boxgrove, Boxgrove Rd, SE2	860	500- 1750
Paddington Green, Park Place Village W2	740	520- 1770
St Saviour's, Lewisham High St, SE13	710	300- 1230
Parliament Hill, Highgate Rd, NW5	700	410- 980
Our Lady's Convent, Amhurst Park N16	660	150- 1410
Brockley, Beecroft Rd, SE4	520	50- 630
George Eliot, Marlborough Hill NW8	510	370- 790
Beechcroft, Beechcroft Rd, SW17	500	130- 970
St Patrick's, Dundee St, E1	510	180- 980
Robert Browning, King & Queen St, SE17	410	80- 760
Rosendale, Turney Rd, SE21	380	210- 940
Rotherhithe, Rotherhithe New Rd, SE16	370	50- 630
St Bernadette, Atkins Rd, SW12	150	60- 230

Four of the schools *had* been specially chosen for the survey because they were situated close to industrial works using lead—Harbinger (3,150ppm), Redriff (1,100), Seven Mills (890) and Boxgrove (860). The rest were chosen at random. Thus 19 schools of those randomly picked breached the 500 'safety level' for no immediately identifiable reason.

Several were on or close to busy roads—suggesting to the survey team that the pollution came from petrol fumes. But the two schools with the highest lead pollution—Telferscot and Rushmore—were 'close to neither a main road nor any known lead works'.

The survey report says: 'This...suggests that sources other than traffic or lead works are sometimes important. There is, however, no doubt that petrol-derived lead is in general the major contributor to lead in urban dust.' It concludes:

> It must be remembered that the 28 schools in this survey are only a small fraction of the total number (1,166) of ILEA schools. The four schools found to warrant further investigation represent, on a simple pro-rata basis, more than 150 schools in the whole of the ILEA area. It is difficult to avoid the conclusion that an ILEA-wide survey should be undertaken.

It was also difficult to persuade ILEA to act decisively. Apart from calling on the Government to reduce lead levels in petrol, little was done in response to the survey report.

Many schools were uncertain whether they had been surveyed for lead or not. Surveyed schools were not told of the results. Only Telferscot was earmarked for follow-up tests because of its high readings. The Telferscot head was told his school was being retested because the school's name 'was drawn out of a hat' and not because it was the most polluted school in the survey. At a parents' meeting called at the school to discuss the pollution, ILEA officials offered to have the children tested for lead poisoning if the parents wished it. This offer was subsequently withdrawn; one reason being that the area health authority said it could not cope with that number of tests. Also, of course, to offer Telferscot children lead-tests would have created the risk that ILEA would have to offer such tests to all London's schoolchildren.

In addition, a letter sent to parents by the Telferscot head—but compiled by ILEA officials—declared:

> Dear Parent
> You may have seen in the Press reports that dust samples taken from the playground at Telferscot School have shown a rather high lead content.
> I have been assured that there is no cause for concern...

The letter was sent to parents 'to stop them panicking until after a meeting with the ILEA officials'. That meeting was demanded by the parents themselves.

The follow-up survey of Telferscot was completed by September 1981. It failed to find the cause of the lead pollution. The readings were below the 5,000 mark recorded in the first survey. The report merely suggested possible causes such as flakes of old leaded paint from a recent redecoration of the school, or 'fall-out' from car maintenance evening classes held at the school. Another suggestion was that the lead came from repainting the school fencing. An unpublished survey of 98 Lambeth public playgrounds, carried out in early 1981 by Lambeth council, had found that a total of 35 per cent of the fencing and play equipment was covered in paint with a lead content more than double the current 'safety limit'. The action so far taken by ILEA and the GLC over lead pollution in schools is to initiate further tests in school playgrounds and to attend meetings at high-risk schools to try to allay parents' fears.

At the same time as ILEA/GLC committees were debating the secret results of the 28 schools survey, the GLC was on the point of adopting an 'action level' for lead in street dust of 5,000ppm, below which it would not act to reduce areas of lead pollution.

Oddly, the GLC criteria for assessing contaminated development land includes a lead level of between 1,000 and 2,000ppm as 'contaminated' and between 2,000 and 10,000ppm as 'heavily contaminated'. On that basis, most of inner London's school playgrounds are contaminated areas.

In 1977, two members of the GLC's own Environmental Sciences Group had declared that 'the hazard from lead in dust has been relatively neglected...in recent years'. In a study of the risk from lead in street dust[1], they noted that to keep within the maximum permissible daily intake of lead in ingested dust, the concentration of lead in street dust should not exceed 300ppm.

The GLC has a massive problem—and admits it. Concentrations of lead in dust of 1,000 to 2,000ppm are typical for the pavements of inner London streets, and it is not unusual to find values of 3,000 to 4,000ppm on the pavements of busy streets.

GLC officials admitted that 5,000ppm was 'clearly not satisfactory in the long term'. But they said it was pointless to adopt a lower level for action since 'the main source of lead in street dust is from lead in petrol'. And that—so far as the GLC and ILEA are concerned—is the Government's business. The GLC argued that 'at least when the level goes over 5,000ppm at any place we will know it must be due to something other than motor exhausts'.

In effect, the GLC was fixing a limit so high that it would rarely have to take *any* action to reduce pollution.

The recommendations for a 5,000ppm 'action' level were rejected following the as yet 'anonymous' GLC school playgrounds survey. On 31 March 1981, new guidelines 'for the assessment of lead pollution' were adopted by the GLC: 500ppm for lead in surface dust, and 1 micro-

---

1. 'Lead in dust in city streets' by M J Duggan and S Williams (*The Science of the Total Environment*, 7, 1977, pp91-97)

gramme of lead per cubic metre of air $(1ug/m^3)$ for airborne lead.

The guidelines, said the Council, 'will be of value in helping to ensure a positive and consistent approach by the Council to those steps it can take to reduce lead pollution'. A joint report by two GLC committees points out:

> However, the guidelines are not attainable at present in many places in London and will continue to be exceeded while some 800 tonnes of lead a year are discharged from motor vehicles in London. The problem is particularly acute on and around heavily-trafficked and often congested major roads which are generally the most densely populated and intensely used by shoppers and pedestrians.[2]

Urban lead pollution is ubiquitous. It gets everywhere—not just into schools. Any street can be affected whether it is a busy main road or a quiet residential side street. Telferscot school is in just such a street. But pollution in schools causes particular concern because children spend a good deal of time in them—and schools are expected to be safe for children. Many schools are not.

In the past, schools have been decorated with paint containing a large amount of lead. Many city schools are sited beside busy roads. Some are near to lead-based industrial plants and smelters. Old paint peels and flakes and gets into the dust of the school and playground: dust already laden with lead particles from car exhausts and industrial fumes.

Sometimes, planning decisions seem particularly perverse. For example, a nursery centre has recently been built next to the Westway motorway in Kensington & Chelsea having been given the go-ahead by one of the government's expert medical advisers—even though survey readings for lead in the air were near to and on some occasions above the recommended safety limits. And the younger the child the more damaging lead pollution can be.

Schools are usually included in city lead surveys—often with the same worrying results as the London survey produced. In 1978, a special DoE survey in Birmingham was conducted around the M6/A38(M) Gravelly Hill interchange—Spaghetti Junction. School playgrounds were included in the area surveyed. The report concluded that the survey 'gave reassuring results... and no child was found with a blood lead level greater than 35ug/100ml'. That's within the supposedly safe limit for children. But at least one member of the survey team disagreed. Dr Robert Stephens of Birmingham University believes the readings were badly misinterpreted. He considered then that some 20 per cent of inner Birmingham children under 13 years of age probably have a lead-induced disturbance of the nervous system. Even this is now reckoned far too low an estimate.

---

2. The report came from the Recreation and Community Services Policy Committee and the Planning and Communications Policy Committee, dated 16 February and 11 March 1981.

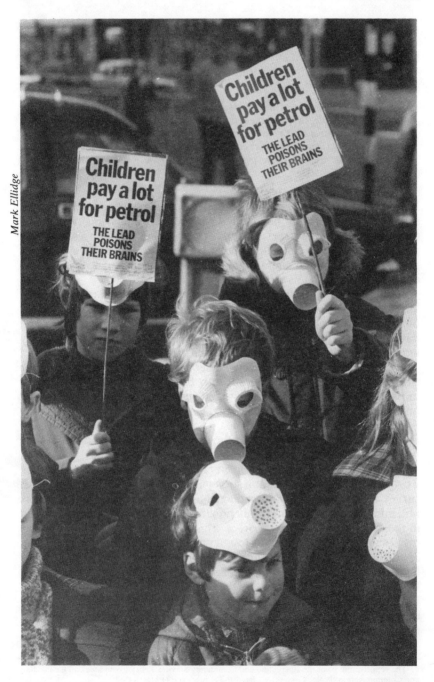

Lead as a pollutant

LEAD is poisonous; it can harm people and it can kill. It is a neuro-toxin—in other words, a brain poison.

Its toxic nature was well known by the second century BC. Lead poisoning was common among the Roman population because they used lead for water pipes and for storing wine. It also became common among industrial workers in Britain during the 19th and early 20th century. In 1905 *Pannell's Reference Book for Home and Office* stated:

> Lead poisoning is of frequent occurrence amongst workers in white or red lead and also in metallic lead. Lead has been known to contaminate drinking water, aerated waters, food wrapped in tin foil, and cider or beer that has been allowed to stand in lead pipes. Lead salts have caused poisons by their presence in drinking water (owing to red lead used in jointing the pipes), as also in hair dye, confectionery (lead chromate being used instead of saffron), dripping preserved in lead-glazed vessels, and even in lead-glazed lining in hats.

It recommended as an antidote to lead poisoning: 'Egg and milk, brandy, and warmth to the abdomen.'

A broad spread of workers were vulnerable to lead poisoning—house painters, plumbers, fitters, accumulator workers, iron plate enamellers, white lead makers, chrome workers, japanners and glaziers, file cutters, compositors and the cappers of bottles. They were assumed to absorb lead in three ways: from contamination of food eaten at the work place, by inhalation of fine lead dust, and by absorption through the skin as the acid sweat dissolved lead dust. Again, advice on 'avoiding lead poisoning' was slight—'a daily bath, cleaning hands before meals (if soiled by lead compounds, with turpentine), and the use of Epsom salts to keep the bowels freely open'.

Since then, the incidence of 'clinical' lead poisoning with obvious and overt symptoms of illness—domestic and industrial—has declined dramatically through improved safety and hygiene measures. For example, in 1977-78, according to Health and Safety Executive figures, 35 cases of occupational lead poisoning were notified under the Factories Act; one was fatal. (In 1975, 65 children under 14 were admitted to hospital with lead poisoning.)

Between 1975 and 1978, 11 per cent of the workers examined by the Employment Medical Advisory Service (EMAS) were found to be over the 80ug/100ml limit. At that time there was only a voluntary agreement of a 'danger' limit of 100ug/100ml, although workers tended to be suspended from work below that level. No accurate statistics are available of the number actually suspended. The Health and Safety Executive (HSE) reckons that just over 800 were taken off work given that some 8,000 workers were officially covered by the voluntary agreement.

New regulations in operation from August 1981 (Control of Lead at Work Regulations 1980) put a statutory danger limit at 80ug/100ml. An additional 2,000 workers are covered by the regulations and HSE estimates that up to 1,000 workers are likely to be suspended at any one time for having elevated lead levels.

However, dangers persist largely because we are being damaged by lead in ways that are subtler and previously unlooked for. The main concern now is not so much with the lethal nature of lead, rather it is the sub-clinical effects that are most universally dangerous. Severe damage can be done, especially to children, at low levels of lead pollution and before any obvious symptoms of poisoning start to show. And while leaded paint is reckoned the most common cause of *clinical* lead poisoning in children, leaded petrol is the main cause of these widespread sub-clinical effects—undercover poisoning.

In addition there is more lead in the environment. The level of airborne lead has been growing steadily—due mainly to the 20th century innovation of adding lead to petrol.

In 1921, an industrial chemist in the USA discovered the organolead anti-knock additive, tetra-ethyl lead (TEL). By 1923, it was being commercially produced by the Ethyl Corporation. In those two years, 139 chemists and workers had been either injured, killed or gone mad from handling TEL. A few drops of pure TEL on the hand are enough to turn someone insane or to kill. TEL was one of the compounds recommended by the CIA to its agents for assassinations. Yet the profitability of this form of improving car engine performance overcame any worries about the effects of lead on workers and on the general environment. Better safety measures were developed, but the continuing dangers were suppressed.

Leaded petrol thus became a major pollutant—and now accounts for some 95 per cent of the lead content of the air. In 1978, an environmental pollution report from the Department of the Environment (DoE) stated:

...emissions of pollutants such as lead, carbon monoxides, hydrocarbons and oxides of nitrogen from petrol engines rose by about 20 per cent in the six years 1970 to 1976[1].

Contemporary urban dwellers have to cope with a uniquely high level of lead inside them. In 1965, an American scientist Clair C Patterson concluded that the amount of lead that humans carried around in their bodies (their body lead burden) that was considered 'normal' is in reality grossly elevated over the 'natural' levels with which the human species evolved. He concluded the modern lead burdens were a toxic insult which might endanger public health. He also identified leaded petrol emissions as a major contributor to those body burdens.

The same conclusion had been reached in the USSR some years before—and leaded petrol had been banned as early as 1959.

A Harvard University study (1979) found that the level of lead in humans in the USA and the UK is 500 times greater than that in the bones of Peruvians who died 1,600 years ago.

A useful yardstick is that in a natural uncontaminated environment, an adult man is estimated to have a natural blood lead level of 0.002 parts per million (ppm), and a total body burden of 2 milligrams of lead or less. But the typical blood lead level of urban man is reckoned at 0.2ppm, with a total body burden of 200 milligrams.

---

1. Digest of environmental pollution statistics (HMSO)

What lead does to us

LEAD damages the central nervous system, brain, heart and kidneys. It can cause anaemia, high blood pressure, abdominal and muscular pains, lethargy and hallucination, abortion and stillbirth. When the level of lead in a child's blood exceeds 80 micrograms of lead per 100 millilitres of blood (80ug/100ml) fits, encephalopathy (inflammation of the brain) and death can occur.

Children are especially vulnerable to the effects of lead because their brain and nervous system are still developing. They also absorb lead more quickly and easily than adults—about five times more. Once the lead is there, it is more difficult to get rid of. The effect is cumulative. Thus children are 'poisoned' at levels lower than adults.

The majority of urban children have lead readings of between 10 and 30 ug/100ml. The most recent study of city children done in the UK showed a range between 7 and 32 ug/100ml. Countries differ over the level of lead in the blood that is acceptable as 'normal' for adults and children. An EEC directive on biological screening of the population for lead has an upper limit of normality for children of 35ug/100ml. But since the 1960s, normal limits have been steadily revised downwards in the USA. The United States Environmental Protection Agency now recommends that the mean blood lead level of children should not exceed 15ug/100ml.

In Britain, doctors and scientists usually talk of 'raised' blood lead levels when those levels register between 30 and 40ug/100ml. However, Derek Bryce-Smith, professor of organic chemistry at Reading University, has stated that 'it is difficult to obtain suitable treatment in this country for children having blood lead levels less than 40ug/100ml in view of the widespread but erroneous belief that a threshold of effect exists and that no child is at risk if the blood lead level is below 40ug/100ml'.

This is the nub of the current argument: at what level does the intake of lead begin to harm people—and children in particular?

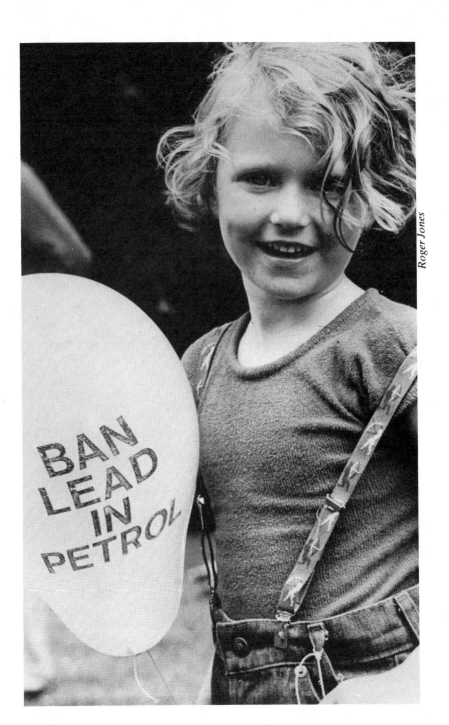

The evidence is growing that a threshold level of lead—a point at which harm starts being done—does not exist. Rather, the effect is a continuum, causing harm at very low levels—well before clinical symptoms of poisoning appear.

For children, these lower level effects include hyperactivity, an inability to concentrate, learning difficulties, psychological and behavioural disturbances. One crucial effect can be a lowered IQ—a potential drop of up to 7 IQ points, sufficient to more than double the number of children in Britain considered mentally retarded. Pre-school children and foetuses in pregnant women are reckoned to be especially vulnerable to these low-level effects.

Thus, it can be said that there is no real evidence for a 'safe' level for lead in the body. And if there is such a level, it is well below the lowest levels now usually found in humans.

The 'safety' limits

A VARIETY of health and environmental agencies set out recommended safety levels for lead in people and in the environment. These are not necessarily statutory. Different agencies sometimes set different safety levels. For example, USA levels are normally lower—ie. more stringent—than those in the UK and the European Commission. The UK now takes its lead safety levels mainly from the Commission.

A 1977 EEC directive has required a systematic population screening programme for lead pollution. The first programme for the UK has recently been completed and published[1]. The second is now underway. The EEC directive sets down 'reference levels' for each group of people surveyed:

> No more than 2 per cent should have a blood lead level over 35ug/100ml; no more than 10 per cent over 30ug/100ml; and no more than 50 per cent over 20ug/100ml.

The Commission must be informed if these levels are exceeded and action taken to trace and reduce the source of the exposure. Several groups, surveyed in the UK as part of the EEC screening programme and in related DoE studies, have breached the EEC reference levels—pregnant women and mothers with young babies in soft water areas, children of lead workers, and children living near busy roads.

The EEC reference levels have no scientific basis. They are based on political criteria which, it was thought, would accommodate virtually all non-industrially exposed populations in the EEC, and thereby provide quasi-scientific public reassurance.

'Safety' levels are also provided for lead in the air, in water, food, dust

---

1. European Community screening programme for lead: United Kingdom results 1979-80 (DoE Pollution Report 10, HMSO, 1981)

and paint, as well as for blood lead levels (or concentrations) in adults and children.

Although blood is most frequently used to assess someone's lead level, blood only gives a reading on current lead absorption. It is not a reliable indicator of past absorption or total body burden of lead. A child's blood lead level will rise and fall depending on how recently the child has been exposed to lead, and how high that exposure was. Tooth or dentine samples give a much more reliable indication of exposure to lead and over a much longer period of time (months rather than days)—past as well as current absorption of lead can be recorded.

People absorb lead in different ways and at different rates. For example, it has been estimated that for each 1,000ppm of lead in dust to which a child is exposed, that child's blood lead increases by 5ug/100ml. However, this figure is subject to wide variations and is critically dependent on the initial blood lead level. For just how much lead a child actually takes in and retains will depend on each child's habits and activities and how much lead is already in a child's body (the higher the existing body level, the smaller the rise produced by each subsequent dose; the lower the level, the more vulnerable a child to each new dose)[2].

Such 'safety' levels are gradually being revised downwards as experts come, officially, to accept the findings of new evidence. What the 'safety' levels still fail to take into account is the danger from low levels of lead in children.

Safety measures for industry are more stringent and monitored more closely than at-risk environments for children. The toxic quality of lead can be gauged from occupational lead poisoning statistics. Male workers are temporarily suspended from work when their blood lead level is 80ug/100ml. Before August 1981, the level was 100ug/100ml. For women 'of reproductive capacity' the level has been reduced to 40ug/100ml. Implementation of this much-needed reform had been delayed for two years.

In recent years, only one male worker has died from lead poisoning while working on lead-based industrial processes. But more children suffer from lead poisoning each year than lead-industry workers—and more die.

A case of actual clinical poisoning will, generally, make a local authority or health authority move fast to locate the source. Indeed, they are obliged to act when blood lead levels in adults and children exceed certain limits. However, where governments and authorities are tardy is in eliminating major pollution sources when no case of *clinical* lead poisoning—with obvious and overt symptoms—has occurred. For example, if a

---

2. Scientists talk about lead intake and lead uptake. *Intake* refers to the amount of lead ingested, breathed in or generally taken on board by the human body; *Uptake* is the amount actually retained in the body tissues, since not all ingested lead is retained. About 55 per cent of inhaled lead is deposited in the lungs and of this nearly all is absorbed.

Workers on industrial injury benefit due to lead poisoning		Hospital admissions for lead poisoning of children under 15	
1974-5	44	1974	50
1975-6	51	1975	50
1976-7	25	1976	50
1977-8	27	1977	80
1978-9	24	1978	70
	171		300

(Social security statistics)   (DHSS statistics)
Between 1968 and 1978, seventeen children under 14 died from some form of lead poisoning (OPCS statistics).

child chews a piece of peeling paint that has a high lead content—say, off a shed in a school playground, that child will begin to show clear signs of lead poisoning: vomiting, extreme lethargy, severe headaches, perhaps even hallucination. Once confirmed, the health authority would be obliged to act to trace and get rid of the lead source. However, a group of children living and going to school in a heavily trafficked area might be registering high blood lead levels, but not officially too high nor showing overt signs of poisoning. They would probably show sub-clinical effects of lead poisoning, if they were able to get a doctor or hospital to carry out tests—and even then there would be a reluctance to link the effects with lead. These children would almost certainly be underachieving educationally and suffering behaviour difficulties. They would experience an IQ loss, and some may even suffer brain damage.

Yet officially they would not be regarded as victims of lead poisoning. Nothing would be done, except perhaps some monitoring of lead pollution along a few of the area's main roads by a sceptical and largely uninterested environmental health department.

Many hospitals and doctors refuse to take blood or even dentine tests on children to check for high lead levels. The British Medical Association (BMA) discourages what it terms 'presymptomatic screening programmes'. It has cited the testing of adults and children to establish their body lead level as an example of the kind of screening that should not be encouraged. The BMA's latest handbook on a medical code of ethics (issued in 1981) puts such screening in the category of 'ethical dilemmas'—although there would appear to be some financial dilemmas in there too. It deserves to be quoted at length.

Screening
5.2 Presymptomatic screening involves a departure from the traditional doctor-patient relationship and therefore has ethical implications. Has the medical

profession any responsibility for 'discovering' illness as distinct from respond-
ing to it when it presents itself? People believing themselves to be ill and
presenting for treatment are only a proportion of the ill people within the
community. Some are unwell but do not seek medical help: others do not know
that they are ill. The ethical dilemma lies in the fact that screening could reveal
many sick persons who do not at present seek medical help.

5.3 Before embarking on a screening programme (other than as a research
procedure) a doctor must satisfy himself that:

    (a) the individuals in a given population wish to know whether they have the
disease for which the screening is proposed.

    (b) the screening techniques he will use are reliable and will not give an
unacceptable level of false negatives or false positives.

    (c) medical science has the ability, and the population, the financial
resources, to provide such practical assistance as is currently available.

5.4 In considering the financial implications the doctor should remember that it
will be some time before the cost of the screening programme is offset by the
benefits accrued from earlier diagnosis of the disease.

In consequence, it is extremely difficult for parents to find out just what
degree of lead burden their children are having to tolerate. The medical
profession, in general, regards such parents as a nuisance, unstable and
liable to panic. On the publication of the DHSS-commissioned Lawther
Report on *Lead and health* in March 1980, the Chief Medical Officer at
the DHSS, Sir Henry Yellowlees, sent out a confidential letter (CMO
(80)8) to all Medical Offficers and Chief Environmental Health Officers
advising them, reluctantly, that they had better prepare for these panicking parents:

    ...the report may attract considerable publicity and some anxiety may be
expected in areas subject to lead pollution. There may be requests for blood
lead estimations in individuals, particularly in children where there is the
possibility of unusual exposure.

    Existing facilities should be sufficient to meet increased demand for blood
lead estimations. It is possible that requests may initially overload local
resources in some areas, and it will be for heads of the local chemical pathology
departments to make appropriate arrangements for carrying out tests to avoid
disrupting existing services.

This letter raises at least one intriguing point. It would seem that the
health authorities are only prepared to offer readily to hand testing
facilities when they fear the populace is near to hysteria. In 'normal'
times, they vigorously discourage the use of such testing by commonsense
and responsible parents concerned for their children.

More sensibly, the BMA prefers doctors to take tooth samples for lead
readings both because this causes less intrusion on the child and is a more
reliable method for finding lead levels in the human body. For these
reasons, the BMA considers the Needleman study (see page 51) 'a
superb and classic piece of work'.

A lead study currently underway in London boroughs is using tooth samples. The study is sponsored by the Department of the Environment to check 'the relationship between body lead levels, behaviour and intelligence in children aged 6 to 8'. Children in Enfield, Hounslow, Kensington and Chelsea, and Hammersmith and Fulham (which includes the Talgarth Road, the most lead-polluted street in Europe) are being checked. Preliminary tests had been made on children in Hammersmith during early 1981, without their parents' knowledge.

Last summer, all the children handed in at school any teeth which fell out over a specified period. Every child got a badge saying 'I gave a tooth'. The lead content of each tooth was measured. Teachers also completed a behaviour rating form for every child handing in a tooth. The form was in three sections: attitude to authority (eg. submissive, defiant, attendance problem); group participation (eg. isolated from other children, no sense of fair play, appears to lack leadership, does not get along with the opposite sex); and classroom behaviour (eg. hums and makes other odd noises, poor co-ordination, overactive, steals).

Of the 2,000-plus seven year olds involved, a special sample of 200 with varying lead levels were given a battery of tests (lasting 1½ hours) on intelligence, academic achievement, reaction time, and visual-motor and auditory performance. Their mothers were also quizzed on each child's medical and educational history, and the conditions in which the child grew up. Parents' attitudes, interest and involvement with the child were also 'explored'. The study should be complete by summer 1982.

Sources of lead pollution

HUMANS absorb lead mainly from food, water and the air. Each source of lead to which someone is exposed helps to build up that person's total body burden of lead. Blood samples reveal the current level of lead in the body; tooth samples the burden carried over a long period of time.

The most common source of lead for humans is generally from the food they eat. However, many people can be exposed to some other, exceptionally high, source—for example, by living near a lead smelting works, or living in a soft-water area in a house with lead plumbing. Such conditions can lift their lead burden over the accepted safety limits.

Children have their own 'high-risk' problems—partly because they absorb lead more readily than adults, and partly because of their habits. Such sources include chewing flaking leaded paint or playing beside busy roads.

Precisely how much lead pollution comes from which sources is a major area of controversy. For example, the proportion of human lead intake from polluted air has been consistently revised upwards—and most of the lead in the air (90 per cent or more) comes from petrol fumes (see page 32).

Lead in food

Food is contaminated by lead in three basic ways: from the soil, from the air, and from containers for storage. The maximum permitted level of lead in most foods is 1 part per million (1ppm), and 0.2ppm for baby food (Lead in Food Regulations 1979, SI 1254, HMSO).

Canned food has a much higher lead content than fresh food because lead-based solders are often used to seal the seams of the cans. There are stringent regulations for canned baby foods. But no warnings are printed on other canned foods that they are unfit for babies and young children. Most amateur pottery glazes contain lead, although commercial pottery is, generally, 'leadfree'. However, the majority of glazes are based on lead. A British Standard specification states that glazes should not release more than 7ppm of lead when tested with dilute acetic acid.

Lead in the soil comes both from lead-rich ores in the ground and—more usually—from lead in the air and in dust. Airborne lead is increasingly regarded as a major source of the pollution of food. Crops, fruit and vegetables grown near busy roads or lead smelters are especially liable to contamination.

Tests show that the level of lead in soil in London is, on average, 500ppm compared with soil in rural areas with an average lead content of only 10 to 20ppm. Local authority environmental health officials frequently test vegetables grown in gardens and allotments near busy roads. Many have an unacceptably high lead content. In 1979, the Mole Valley council in Surrey became the first local authority to test an area for lead pollution *before* a motorway was built. They tested vegetables growing within 25 metres of the proposed M25 extension. The local environmental health officer said that 'if the road is to be built we will need information prior to its completion on lead levels in homegrown vegetables for comparison'. So at least Mole Valley will know by just how much a motorway ups the local lead level.

It is generally accepted by scientists that we absorb the majority of our lead directly from food and drink. But this fact has often been used by some scientists to ignore or reject the serious effects of leaded petrol. The evidence is piling up that food crops derive a growing proportion of lead from petrol fumes.

Two recent investigations have revealed the large-scale increase in crop pollution by petrol fumes (Rabinowitz, 1972), and the contamination of crops by lead some distance from main roads or industrial processes (Tjell, Hovmand & Mosbaek, 1979).

Michael Rabinowitz, writing on his survey in *Chemosphere* (number 4, 1972), concluded that 'if lead were removed from gasoline, there would be an immediate decrease of about 80 per cent in the lead content of crops, with a subsequent decrease in human exposure'.

The Tjell/Hovmand/Mosbaek study in Denmark overthrew the conventional view that crop contamination from airborne lead is of no great significance. That view said such contamination ceased after 100 to 200 metres from the road. The Danish study found that lead in grass in a 'remote' rural area came mainly from the atmosphere. The study was undertaken 5km from any industrial plant and 1km from a main highway (22,000 cars every 24 hours). The area was surrounded by agricultural farmland and forest. It was found that lead from the atmosphere was responsible for 90 to 99 per cent of the total lead content of the grass. In short, lead pollution travels further than was thought.

Scientists at the Atomic Energy Research Establishment at Harwell were so impressed by this study that they have set up a repeat of the research. It is due for completion in 1982.

An early Harwell study in 1978 had concluded that airborne lead dispersed rapidly between 18 and 36 metres. They now admit that the techniques used were inappropriate for establishing long-range effects.

Dr Robert Stephens of Birmingham University points out that: 'Even if only 0.1 per cent of the 7,000 tonnes of lead which are released into the atmosphere from petrol in the UK actually get deposited on food crops, this represents more than the presently accepted annual dietary intake for the whole population.'

Lead in paint

In the late 1960s, a spate of lead poisonings and high lead levels in American children was traced to leaded paint on the walls of homes. It was the beginning of serious doubts over the accepted view on lead pollution—that there was no cause for concern.

> Lead poisoning due to eating of peeling lead paint on dilapidated houses by children with pica had only begun to receive long overdue attention... no-one had suspected that undue lead absorption was so widespread among children. When it was discovered that most of these children had no overt symptoms of poisoning, lead poisoning suddenly became problematic and controversial. (Jane Lin-Fu, *New England Journal of Medicine,* March 1979)

Yet leaded paint remains a major cause of lead poisoning among children both in America and Britain. One recent study in the UK put the proportion at 20 in every 100 cases of clinical lead poisoning. Lead in paint is the most frequent cause of death from lead poisoning.

Children with pica—the condition of eating or ingesting 'substances not normally regarded as foodstuffs'—often chew pieces of flaking or peeling paint. If that paint is heavily leaded, clinical poisoning can occur. However, studies in America show that over 20 per cent of cases of clinical lead poisoning in children have been caused by chewing *intact* rather than peeling paint.

Lead has been added to paint for centuries—first as a key part of the paint making process; now as pigments and drying agents. The use of lead in paint has declined considerably—'leaded' paint makes up an estimated three per cent of current UK sales. But most paints still contain *some* lead from the lead naphthenate used as a drying agent.

In Britain, there are no statutory regulations to limit the level of lead in paint. There exists only a voluntary agreement between government and the paint industry that warning labels be placed on cans of paint with more than 1 per cent of lead (10,000ppm). The industry itself monitors lead levels in paint and the placing of warning labels. But the voluntary nature of the code has been shown to be inadequate. At least one paint company does not conform to the agreement—and a 1972 survey in Birmingham revealed that many high-leaded paints were carrying no warning at all.

In February this year, Geoffrey Lean the *Observer*'s environment correspondent revealed that paint being sold in some supermarkets contained more than 15 times the 'safe' level of lead (15.6 per cent). The cans of paint, made by the London-based firm Rustin's, merely had a label saying 'Contains lead'. The voluntary code between government and the industry's trade association, the Paintmakers Association, proposes the wording: 'Not suitable for use on surfaces liable to be chewed or sucked by children.' Rustin's is not a member of the Association. Managing director, Ronald Rustin, was reported in *The Observer* (14 February 1982) as saying: 'When we produce a product that we think might be harmful, the warning goes on straight away, but we are not convinced that the danger from lead-based paint is as bad as people make out. The people campaigning against lead in petrol have a much stronger case.'

A large amount of old leaded paint remains on Britain's buildings— inside and out. But no figures are available as to the amount still around— and accessible to children. A 1969 survey of part of London found that over half the homes surveyed had leaded paint accessible to children.

'High-risk' painted areas include wooden surfaces—doors, windows, sheds; street furniture, wrought iron, steel structures; playground equipment. Many schools still have old leaded paint on buildings which remain a constant hazard.

A recent survey of playground equipment by Lambeth environmental health department found that 35 per cent of the equipment and nearby railings in a total of 98 public playgrounds were covered in paint with a lead content more than double the current safety limit.

Lead chromate is widely used as a yellow pigment. This is included in the paint for the yellow lines on the roads.

Several countries, such as West Germany, have banned lead-based paint. The USA has a maximum limit of lead in paint of 600ppm or 0.06 per cent—compared with Britain's 10,000ppm.

In 1980, Deansfield primary school playground in Greenwich was being badly polluted by paint with a high lead content flaking off a playground shed. Some of the children's blood lead levels were higher than they should be. The shed was stripped and repainted. Early in 1981, St Patrick's primary school in Plumstead, South-East London, was checked for pollution after a child was diagnosed as having lead poisoning. Greenwich council recommended that areas of the school be repainted and the playground washed down.

A follow-up study[1] of some Greenwich schools, published in January 1982, found that many of them had paint with a lead content substantially higher than is reckoned safe. Only one of the seven schools was found to

---

1. *Environmental Health* magazine (January 1982); see also *The Observer* (17 January 1982).

be 'safe' from leaded paint. Boxgrove had paint with up to 6 per cent lead; Thomas A'Beckett and Alexander McLeod 4.2 per cent; Manormead and De Lucy 1.5 per cent. The authors of the study—environmental health officers—believe that such problems are widespread across Britain.

Ironically, in view of Mr Rustin's comment above, the report's authors maintain that lead in paint is the main source of high lead levels in children and not lead in petrol.

Lead-free paint has been available and advertised in appropriate magazines for many years—in some cases before world war two. However, many local authorities have continued to use high lead paint for its schools and nurseries. A report by the GLC to its, and ILEA's, committees dated April 1980 states:

> In most buildings built before 1970 (and that includes many... ILEA schools), the layers of paint originally applied will have a high lead content. However, these layers of paint may now be covered by new low lead paint. Provided the paint surface remains intact there should be no problem. It is only if such paints deteriorate and flake (thus exposing original layers) that the chance of ingestion by a child arises.

Since 1973 the GLC and ILEA has used paint for top surfaces with a lead content of below one per cent—and, since 1979, also for priming paint. The EEC recommends that paint with a lead content of *0.5 per cent* or above should have a warning label.

A subsequent ILEA report dated March 1981 stated:

> Since the early 1970s, it has been the policy of the Authority to use only low-lead paint and, more recently, low-lead primers. The paint film on surfaces will, therefore, contain lead in varying quantities, but almost all will have been recoated with low-lead paint under the 6-year redecoration cycle. The major proportion of leaded paint is located on joinery (eg. doors, cupboards) rather than on wall surfaces, since emulsion paints do not contain lead.

Nonetheless, there have been regular incidences of children suffering from lead poisoning because of the presence of leaded paint in UK schools, including London.

Lead in water

In December 1980, the *New Statesman* revealed that a Government survey of new-born babies in Glasgow, showing that more than one in ten were born with a blood lead level above the EEC safety level for adults, had been kept secret for over a year. Doctors who worked on the survey, carried out during 1979, claimed that Government ministers and civil servants had been—and still were—hampering the publication of the report.

The high lead levels are due to a combination of the lead piping and tanks used to carry the city's water supply and the very soft water in the area. This makes it easy for lead to transfer from the piping to the water. Before birth, babies receive the lead via the mother's placenta.

The survey was part of an EEC screening programme for lead pollution being carried out under the auspices of the Department of the Environment. It should have been included in the Lawther Report *Lead and*

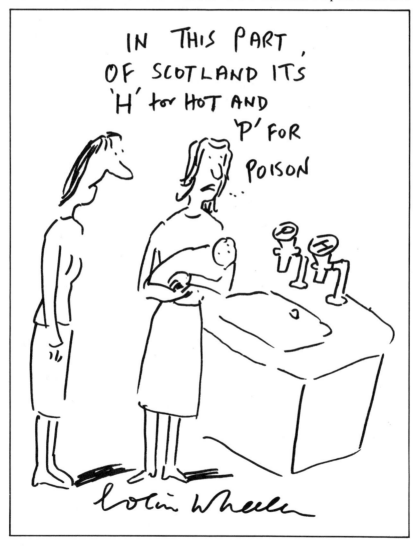

health (March 1980). This played down the effects of lead pollution in children—and failed to consider the issue of lead crossing the mother's placenta to the foetus.

The EEC's recommended blood lead level for adults is 35ug/100ml and suggests a 'safe' level for children of 15ug/100ml. Sixty-two per cent of the Glasgow babies were above the child lead 'norm' of 15ug/100ml. Eleven per cent above the adult safe level of 35ug/100ml. The highest average reading was 51ug/100ml.

Another recent Glasgow study (Moore and Goldberg) measured water lead levels in the homes of 77 mentally retarded children, in whom no cause had been found for their disability, and in the homes of 77 normal children. They also measured the lead in the water of the houses lived in by the mothers during pregnancy. The lead concentration in the water was significantly higher for the mentally retarded group. A child is twice as likely to be mentally retarded if the water lead level in the home during pregnancy or the first year of life is over a limit of 800 milligrammes of lead per litre of water. Many Glasgow homes are above that limit.

Dr Michael Moore, who worked on both surveys, says of the newborn baby study:

> No-one here or abroad has produced such high lead pollution figures for a general population survey. One in 20 of the population is over-exposed in most gross terms. Children are a critical at-risk group.

Neighbourhoods around lead smelters tend to produce lead pollution figures close to those in Glasgow.

Early in 1981, it was discovered that the water supplying the Scottish town of Ayr was badly polluted with lead. Tests on mothers in the town revealed that between 15 to 20 per cent had blood lead levels of over 40ug/100ml—one mother's level was over 60 and another's over 100ug/100ml. (Male workers in the lead industry are suspended from work for health reasons at 80ug/100ml; women workers of childbearing capacity are suspended at 40ug/100ml,)

The babies of these mothers would have the same blood lead levels. All babies under six months were put on a diet of distilled water. A special lime dosing plant was built to reduce the lead content of the water supply. By July 1981, the situation was considered to be under control.

But many other towns in the central area of Scotland—Renfrew is the latest to be identified—are reckoned to be in similar circumstances. It is estimated that in the Strathclyde region there are over 400 danger sources in supplying water that will become heavily polluted from lead in the plumbing systems of the houses.

Lead gets into Britain's water supply mainly from the use of lead for pipes, water tanks and soldered joints. Old buildings are more likely to have lead plumbing. Since 1945, rising costs and a greater awareness of the dangers have curtailed the use of lead. Nonetheless, it is estimated that between 7 and 10.5 million out of the 18.5 million households in

England, Scotland and Wales have lead plumbing.

The lead in the plumbing system dissolves into the water. The lead is transferred to humans by drinking and by using water for preparing and cooking food. The pollution risk is usually much higher in soft-water than in hard-water areas as the lead dissolves more easily.

Out of 5 million households in water-lead problem areas, 2.5 million are reckoned to have lead plumbing. In addition, about 10 per cent of hard-water areas are known to pose problems of lead pollution.

The average amount of lead in Britain's water is 0.02mg per litre, and the average human intake of lead from water is 0.28mg per week. The World Health Organisation (WHO) recommends that a person's weekly intake of lead from all sources should not exceed 3mg. The WHO limit for lead in water for human consumption is 0.1mg per litre. The EEC recommends 0.05mg per litre—and suggests action be taken if the level frequently exceeds 0.1mg. A 1975-6 DoE survey found that 4.3 per cent of British households had a lead level in tap water exceeding the 0.1mg mark.

Three options are available to counteract lead in the water supply. Pipe replacement, flushing at the tap and treating the water at source. To replace lead piping in all 2.5 million 'at risk' households is estimated to cost £1,000 million—two thirds of which would, it is stated by the water industry, be passed on to the consumer. Flushing at the tap relies on each consumer's awareness of the problem—and memory. Flushing for several minutes each time the tap is turned on would increase domestic demand by 17 per cent—and it is doubtful that the water industry could cope with that increase.

Water treatment at source is the industry's preferred option. However, this would be inadequate for many 'high risk' areas, for which pipe replacement is the only solution. The estimated cost for all these areas together is, according to the water industry, £330 million of which £220 million would have to be found by consumers.

In May 1981, the Government announced that people wishing to replace their lead plumbing will be eligible for 50 per cent home improvement grant. However, discussions between the local authorities and the Government over the arrangements for this have been pro-longed—and grants are still unavailable in 1982. Moreover, the total grant-allocation for home improvements was not to be increased to meet the additional demand.

On 17 February 1982, following publication of a DoE diet study of 131 Glasgow mothers and babies, further official action was proposed by the Scottish Secretary of State, George Younger. The study found that high water-lead concentrations were associated with raised dietary lead intakes and blood-leads, particularly for bottle-fed babies. As amounts of ingested lead increased, steadily smaller increases in blood lead were recorded. Use of water from hot taps to make babies' feeds appeared to raise any intakes considerably.

Lime dosing of the city's water supply is being increased. An extra £3 million is now to be made available to Scottish local authorities only for bypassing or replacing lead plumbing. A further £1 million will be spent on surveys of houses likely to have a lead in water problem and on an 'information and education exercise to alert householders... affected by lead in water of the measures they themselves can take to reduce the hazard'. (See *The Glasgow duplicate diet study 1979/80* (Pollution Report No 11, 1982; Department of the Environment). See also House of Commons *Hansard* written answer 17 February 1982, cols 171/2.)

Lead in the air

Food is the most common source of lead for most people. But it is airborne lead that acts as a major contaminator of food crops—and most lead in the air comes from petrol fumes: estimates range between 90 and 99 per cent.

Official thinking on airborne lead has been that human lead intake from the atmosphere is negligible. In September 1977, Kenneth Marks MP, then a DoE Minister stated:

> It is important to realise that airborne lead is unlikely to account for more than a minor proportion of the total lead absorbed into the body... there is no evidence of any hazard to health attributable to lead in exhaust fumes, or to lead in the general environment.

The Government's main source of information on airborne lead has been from the Atomic Energy Research Establishment at Harwell. Most of the research done on lead pollution in the air at Harwell has been funded wholly or in part by the lead and oil industries. A major study between 1974 and 1976, *Human uptake of lead—phase 1,* concluded that humans absorb only 5 per cent of their total lead burden from the air. The report was widely publicised. A second study in 1978, *Human uptake of lead—phase 2,* found that the figure should be 10 per cent—twice as much as previously thought. It was also admitted that in 'hot-spot' areas such as heavy traffic routes or near lead smelters, the figure could be about 50 per cent[2]. The report was kept secret until a copy sent to an American university for research purposes was forwarded to the *Yorkshire Post* in Britain.

A 1974 DoE Pollution Paper *Lead in the environment and its significance to man* stated that lead in the air was a minor contributor to lead in the urban population. Since then there has been a slow reassessment of the role of airborne lead.

---

2. The first study cost £95,600 of which 23 per cent came from member companies of the Institute of Petroleum and the International Lead and Zinc Research Organisation. The second study, published under the title of *Investigations into lead from motor vehicles,* received 32 per cent of its total cost of £119,000 from these sources. See *Hansard,* 29 November 1978, cols 263/4.

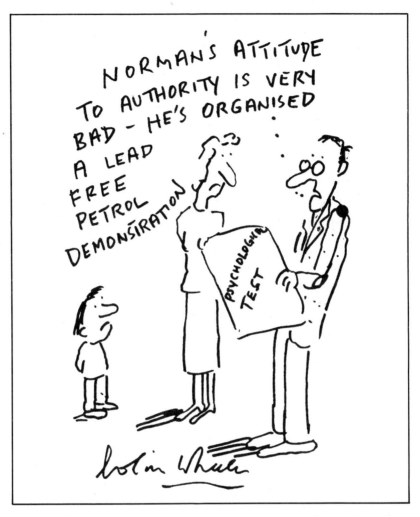

Industrial plants also affect local levels of lead in the air. For example, in 1978, children at the south-east London Boxgrove primary school near a lead smelting works suffered nausea, stomach pains and headaches. Teachers also felt unwell. Two DoE surveys of children at the school in 1972 and 1977 had revealed no abnormal blood lead levels in the children. It was claimed there was no cause for concern. But by July 1978, the Boxgrove head was calling for a public inquiry because of 'an alarmingly high lead pollution level at the school'. Another school in the Abbey Wood area of London was recording dangerously high lead levels in the dust around the school, due partly to the existence of a chloride metal (lead smelting) factory in the area. Levels of 20,000 parts of lead to a million parts of dust (ppm) were recorded. The recommended 'action' level by the EEC, and now by the GLC, is 500ppm.

There is now a greater awareness that airborne lead plays a substantial part in polluting people, especially children. Within three years, the estimates of airborne lead's contribution has jumped from a mere 5 per cent to a broad spread of between 16 and 69 per cent.

Lead in petrol

Between 90 and 99 per cent of the lead in the air comes from petrol fumes. Within 60 years, leaded petrol has become a massive and deeply pervasive pollutant. The immediate consequence of leaded petrol is that between eight and ten thousand tonnes of lead is pushed, or emitted, into Britain's air—as much as 1,000 tonnes in the London area, where a quarter of Britain's traffic operates. The current state of affairs has been succinctly put in the Conservation Society's report *Lead or health*:

> Fall-out of airborne lead from petrol additives is not so much creating a new situation as making an existing situation much worse.
> It cannot be stressed too much that this sort of metal pollution is *permanent*. Once lead pollutes soil, there is no feasible way to remove it. It never decays, and is cumulative in soil, just as in the human body.

Lead is added to petrol at the refining stage by each oil company. The sole

---

Associated Octel

The Associated Ethyl Company was registered as a private company in 1938. In 1961 it changed its name to Associated Octel. It is based at Ellesmere Port, Cheshire, with a registered office in London's Berkeley Square.

Associated Octel is owned jointly by five major oil companies: BP, Shell, Mobil, Chevron and Texaco. It is engaged in the manufacture and sale of anti-knock compounds; the provision of managerial, technical and administrative services; and the leasing of property, plant and equipment. There are subsidiaries in France, West Germany and Italy.

The company employs 2,831 people and has a turnover of £60 million (1979). Net profit before tax in that year was £6.8 million; retained profit £2.2 million. Its net current assets were £11 million with fixed assets of £41 million. Between 1975 and 1979, Associated Octel received government grants totalling over £3.5 million. In 1981, the company received a Queen's Award for Export.

UK manufacturer of lead additives for petrol is Associated Octel, based at Ellesmere Port in Cheshire.

The level of lead added to petrol is regulated by each country. These levels have been steadily reduced over the years. Several countries have banned leaded petrol including Japan, USSR and Australia (from 1985); others offer both leaded and leadfree petrol, as in USA.

Britain has always lagged behind other countries in reducing the amount of lead added to petrol—although it is not any longer among the high leads. The current level is 0.40 grams of lead per litre of petrol (0.40g/l). West Germany has a level of 0.15g/l; the USA 0.13g/l.

It was only in 1972 that Britain decided to drop its level from 0.84 to 0.45g/l 'as a precaution'. It also reached an agreement with the oil companies that total annual lead emissions from car exhausts—the lead coming from the burnt petrol—should not exceed the Government-estimated 1971 level of around 7,500 tonnes. Other estimates have put the total annual lead emission at between 8,000 and 10,000 tonnes. Scientific staff at the Greater London Council estimate that 800 tonnes—and perhaps as much as 1,000 tonnes—falls on London every year. Rising petrol sales meant that the 1971 level would be breached in 1981—one reason for the subsequent drop in the petrol lead level in January 1981 to 0.40g/l; another was the pressure of an EEC directive. Nonetheless, the new limit merely slows the rise in pollution rather than reversing it.

There are several spin-off risks from leaded petrol. Used car dumps, the need to dispose of 2½ million highly-leaded car exhausts each year, and the burning of sump oil all contribute to the pollution of the environment—and of children.

Children are poisoned by leaded petrol in two ways. They pick it up directly from car exhausts—young children are about the same height as the source; and from the dust that settles in urban areas—for city dust is laden with lead particles.

Lead in petrol has a special hazard in that uncombusted lead is organic lead, which is much more poisonous than inorganic lead. Inorganic lead is prevented from reaching the brain by what is known as the blood brain barrier. But organic lead can cross that barrier. In London, there is a high level of exposure to organic lead.

With all these known dangers, the actions of the oil companies often seem deeply perverse. For example, the Mobil Oil Company is planning to launch a series of take-away fastfood units on its filling station forecourts. The first—at the Bush Centre filling station by Shepherd's Bush Green in West London—was approved by Hammersmith and Fulham council's planning department in December 1980. The Council's health department was informed of the Mobil application but, according to a local health official, 'somehow our comments were not sent back to the planning people'.

The Mobil Oil plan has been severely criticised by environmentalists and the anti-lead lobby. Professor Derek Bryce-Smith of Reading Uni-

versity, and co-author of the Conservation Society's critical study of the
Lawther Report, said:

> Petrol and food don't mix. Tests carried out by the Transport and Road
> Research Laboratory show that over 50 per cent of the lead in the atmosphere
> around filling stations is organic lead. And that is acutely more poisonous than
> the more usual inorganic lead.

Studies carried out in New Zealand of dogs living on filling station forecourts have revealed substantial amounts of lead in their bodies—over 40
times more than is normal[3]. Some have died prematurely from lead
poisoning. Such results have persuaded the New Zealand Government to
set up a detailed investigation of lead pollution in the country. Surveys in
Australia have come up with similar findings.

Derek Birtles of Mobil's retailing section said Mobil is the first oil
company in Britain to go into the fastfood business: 'With the energy
crisis and petrol price wars, we need additional profit centres.' Mobil runs
1,300 garages in the UK and is currently negotiating for two more
fastfood units in Warrington and Sheffield.

Birtles said: 'All our food will be cooked in microwave ovens, pack-
aged and untouched by human hand.' Hot dogs, hamburgers, bacon-
burgers and chips are all likely to be offered for sale—plus a special Mobil
'petrolburger'. These are all foods with a high fat content, which tends to
encourage a quicker and easier uptake of lead from the gut. Recent
studies with rats show that eating high-fat foods increases lead uptake by
50 times. Birtles claimed: 'I know nothing at all about leaded petrol. The
lead connection is way above my head. The lead thing is a white ele-
phant.'

Children are major customers of fastfood chains. They are also especially vulnerable to the effects of lead pollution. Putting fastfood outlets on
petrol station forecourts will make a dangerous combination for children.
Shepherd's Bush Green is a key 'staging post' for children travelling to
and from school—on foot, by bike, or changing buses. Six primary
schools are within a short walk of the Green. In those areas of the country
where the school meals service has been cut back, fastfood chains are
attracting children at lunchtimes with special offers.

Other sources of lead pollution

There are numerous other sources of lead which make lead levels in
humans rise and which also cause lead poisoning. These include:

Some eye cosmetics, hair darkening products and medicines imported
from the Indian sub-continent. Most of these are banned by the Cosmetic

---

3. *Lead levels in whole blood of New Zealand domestic animals* by N I Ward *et al* (Massey University, New
Zealand).

Products Regulations 1978, although many products still find their way into Britain. (See *Lead and health*, DHSS, 1980 for a detailed rundown, pages 37-40.)

Some hobbies can produce a lead hazard, such as jewellery and stained glass making, lead shot, fishing weights. Some foreign toys are still decorated with high-leaded paint.

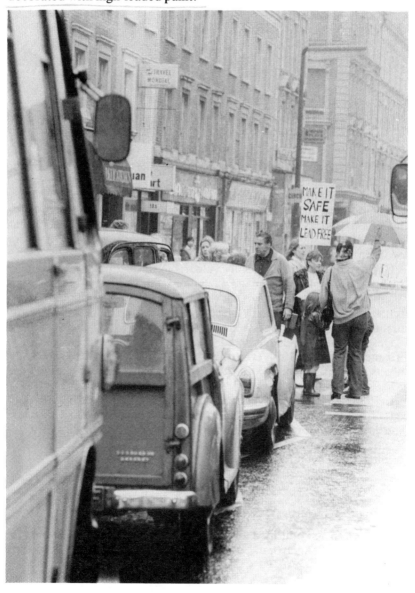

Lead and gypsy children

IN 1979, children on a Greenwich caravan site in South East London were found to have blood lead levels above the UK norm. High levels of lead and another poison, cadmium, were also recorded on the site. These had come from the car fragments and domestic appliances collected on the site to sell as scrap. A 1978 Harwell study of West London had concluded that metal scrapyards were 'extremely significant' in raising local lead levels.

Gypsy children are especially vulnerable to lead pollution. Many of their parents deal in scrap metal, including lead. They often have to live in an environment that contains car dumps and sump oil burning. In addition, local authorities usually place travellers' sites on derelict and frequently contaminated land, and next to busy roads.

Despite the well-documented dangers, scrapyards are outside the jurisdiction of the 1974 Control of Pollution Act—and that in effect means there is no control on the 2½ million dangerously polluted car exhausts thrown away each year.

In 1980, the Westway gypsy caravan site was investigated by a research team from the Westminster Medical School at the request of a local GP. The land was found to be 'heavily contaminated' according to GLC criteria. Blood lead tests were carried out on 23 of the children. The research team's report states:

> Only four children had blood lead levels less than or equal to 20ug/100ml, 13 had blood levels between 21 and 30 and the other 6 children had blood lead concentrations greater than 35ug/100ml, four of these being over 40.

Subsequent tests confirmed that 25 per cent of the children were over the 'safe' limit of 35ug/100ml. Some were showing signs of low lead level poisoning.

The two councils responsible for the site—Hammersmith & Fulham and Kensington & Chelsea—rejected the investigation as 'invalidated', even though their own tests were showing similar results. In August 1981, the North Kensington law centre took the two councils to court under the Public Health Act 1936 in an attempt to get the site relocated.

The law centre lost the case on the grounds that the gypsies had contributed to the poor state of the site and therefore the councils were absolved of responsibility. As for the children's high lead levels, these were considered to be the responsibility of central government because only it had the power to eliminate lead from petrol. But for years successive governments have been very reluctant to do anything about lead in petrol.

The Lawther Report

IN NOVEMBER 1978, the Department of Health and Social Security set up a working party of 12 scientists under Professor Patrick Lawther to consider the question of lead pollution. Its terms of reference were 'to review the overall effects on health of environmental lead from all sources and, in particular, its effects on the health and development of children and to assess the contribution lead in petrol makes to the body burden'.

The composition of that working party was unfortunate. It was weighted towards the scientific view that lead in petrol is of minor importance as a pollutant, and also against the view that 'normal' lead levels in children might have harmful effects. For example, a 1974 study by two of its members, Dr Richard Lansdown and Dr Barbara Clayton, on blood lead levels in children concluded that 'lower levels of intelligence and higher rates of disturbance were found to be more related to social factors'[1].

Several members declared a pecuniary interest to DHSS officials, mainly through consultancies with the lead and oil industries. Some had had research work funded by these industries, although the members declared that the work had always been assessed and published independently of the industries. For example, Dr Donald Barltrop had had research work funded by the International Lead and Zinc Research Organisation.

---

1. *Blood lead levels, behaviour and intelligence: a population study* (The Lancet, 30 March 1974) The report was summarised: 'The total population of children under the age of 17 living in a working class area exposed to undue amounts of lead was examined in an investigation of the relationship between blood-lead levels, general intelligence, reading ability, and rate of behaviour disorder. Distance from the factory producing the lead pollution was related to blood-lead level, but there was no relationship between blood-lead level and any measure of mental functioning. Lower levels of intelligence and higher rates of disturbance were found to be more related to social factors'.

> The 12 experts were: Professor P J Lawther, Professor of Environmental and Preventive Medicine at St Bartholomew's Hospital Medical College, University of London, and head of the clinical section of the Medical Research Council's toxicology unit.
>
> Dr D Barltrop, Director of the Child Health Department at Westminster Children's Hospital, London.
>
> Dr R M Chamberlain, senior epidemiologist at the Central Public Health Laboratory, London.
>
> Professor B E Clayton, Professor of Chemical Pathology and Human Metabolism at the University of Southampton.
>
> Professor W W Holland, Professor of Clinical Epidemiology and Social Medicines at St Thomas' Hospital Medical School, University of London.
>
> Dr R G Lansdown, Principal Psychologist at the Department of Psychological Medicine, Hospital for Sick Children, London.
>
> Dr B Moore, Honorary Research Fellow at the Department of Mathematical Statistics and Operational Research, University of Exeter.
>
> Professor T E Oppe, Professor of Paediatrics at St Mary's Hospital Medical School, University of London.
>
> Professor M Rutter, Professor of Child Psychiatry at the Institute of Psychiatry, University of London.
>
> Dr H A Waldron, Senior Lecturer in Occupational Medicine at the London School of Hygiene and Tropical Medicine, University of London.
>
> Mr R E Waller, Member of MRC Scientific Staff, St Bartholomew's Hospital Medical College, University of London.
>
> Dr W Yule, Senior Lecturer in Psychology at the Institute of Psychiatry, University of London.

Dr Barltrop had also given evidence on behalf of the lead industry in Canada, and in 1981 planned to do so on behalf of the oil industry in Idaho. His stance on the lead issue caused a problem at the start of the working party's deliberations. At the end of November 1978, he had prepared an affidavit on behalf of BP, Shell and Associated Octel for a court case brought by some London parents alleging harm to their children from lead in petrol. Dr Barltrop's action led to him being opposed as an expert witness in an enquiry into the building of the M25. The enquiry inspector agreed that it was important for witnesses to be seen as independent and acceptable to both sides in the enquiry and refused to hear Dr Barltrop. (After questions in the Commons, he was subsequently invited back to the enquiry because the inspector 'did not intend to cast doubt on Dr Barltrop's professional integrity'.)

One Lawther expert was in the process of moving away from the view that lead in petrol was hazardous. Dr Tony Waldron had in the early 1970s been involved with several studies showing evidence of the link between blood lead levels and air lead levels (made up largely from petrol lead)[2]. He subsequently moved from a post in Birmingham to the London School of Hygiene and Tropical Medicine, an institution known to be antagonistic to the argument against leaded petrol. Dr Waldron's work now leads him to regard lead in petrol to be as 'toxicologically significant as a gnat farting in the Albert Hall'[3].

The report of the Lawther working party was published on 28 March 1980 under the title *Lead and health*. It is a detailed but deeply flawed document. For it played down the damaging effects of leaded petrol and called for more research before any concerted action was to be taken. Energies, declared the report, should rather be put into eliminating the 'incontrovertible' sources of lead pollution, such as lead in paint and in water.

On the plus side, it did provide a fairly comprehensive survey of most of the lead hazards—food, tap water, paint, imported cosmetics—backed by some useful, though at times inconsistent, documentation and statistics. But its 'recommendations for action' even in these areas were curiously restrained. For example, the report highlighted the danger from lead in paint. Indeed, several working party members consider it the most dangerous source of lead pollution in children. Yet they failed to recommend the abolition of the inadequate voluntary code between industry and government for controlling lead in paint in favour of statutory regulations. They merely suggested that:

> The lead content of all paint available for retail sale, including paint intended for the exterior surfaces of houses and for institutions, schools and play areas should be as low as is technically feasible.

More seriously, the tenor of the report as a whole was to steer people, intentionally or otherwise, away from lead in petrol as a major threat to the wellbeing of children. The report contains six fundamental errors.
1. It underestimated the contribution of lead-rich dust to the total lead intake of children, and rejected the evidence of the Billick study of New York children showing that their blood lead levels rose and fell in direct relation to the rise and fall in the amount of leaded petrol sold and subsequently combusted into the city air. (Blood lead levels go up and down according to current lead exposure.)
2. It rejected the possibility that atmospheric lead (derived mostly from leaded petrol) might contribute significantly to the amount of lead in food. The working party claimed to 'have seen no evidence that this is

---

2. For example, see *Nature* (253, 345, 1975) Lead levels in blood of residents near the M6-A38(M) interchange, Birmingham.

3. Reported in *Medical News* 25 June 1981.

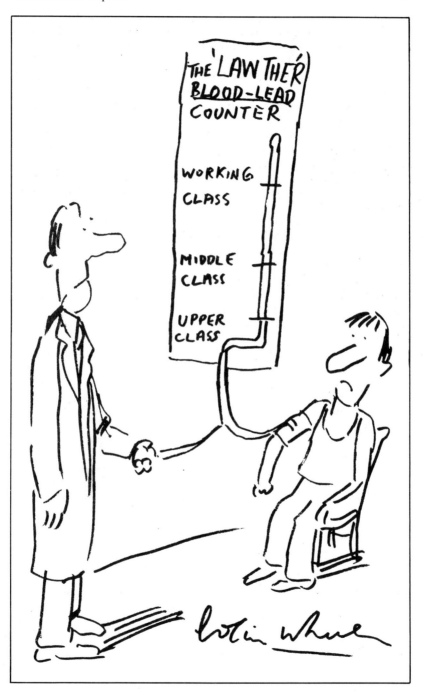

substantially enhanced by contamination by airborne lead'. Examples of such evidence, unseen or ignored by the 12 scientists, include the Danish study of Tjell, Hovmand and Mosbaek (1979) which found that lead from the air was responsible for 90 to 99 per cent of the total lead content in grass in rural areas; and a Reading environmental health department study (1978) which revealed that the lead content of the outer leaves of cabbages was greater by a ratio of 10:1 than the content of the inner leaves.

3. It overestimated the contribution of food and water towards human lead intake. The working party calculated that these two account for 84 per cent of such intake, with air—and thus leaded petrol—taking up just 16 per cent. But evidence, based in part on Government departmental statistics and not discussed by the working party, has put lead intake from the air at between 32 and 69 per cent[4].

4. It ignored or rejected the evidence of highly respected studies from abroad, notably the 1979 Needleman study, that link exposure to leaded petrol with detrimental effects on 'the intelligence, behaviour and performance of children'.

5. It did not consider at all the growing body of biochemical evidence that lead can cause structural and chemical changes in the brain, which affect both behaviour and learning ability[5].

6. It failed to discuss the issue of foetal damage caused by lead crossing the mother's placenta. Several studies[6] have found that the lead levels in stillborn and malformed babies are elevated above the normal level—in some cases 5 to 10 times above the norm. There is also evidence that lead tends significantly to encourage premature birth[7].

In 1977, D G Wibberley found that only 7 per cent of normal births had placental lead levels above 1.5 ug/dl whereas more than 60 per cent of stillbirths or neonatal deaths had levels above this. In 1979, studies by Dr Fraser Alexander in Newcastle 'suggested that throughout pregnancy

---

4. See *The health effects of lead on children* (Conservation Society, 1978); D Bryce-Smith, R Stephens and J Matthews in *Ambio* 7, 1978, page 192; *Lead or health* (Conservation Society, 1980, pages 32-36; and Ministry of Agriculture, Fisheries and Food Statistics, 1980.

5. 'We... have a large body of evidence that 'low-level' lead interferes with numerous important chemical mechanisms involved in the brain's maturation, its neurotransmitter metabolism, the regulation of its energy supplies, its mediation of sensory inputs, and its behavioural outputs. None of these matters are mentioned in the Lawther Report.' (Prof D Bryce-Smith and Dr R Stephens in *Lead or health*).

6. For example: see D Bryce-Smith, R R Deshpande, J Hughes & H A Waldron (The Lancet, 1977, i, 1159); D G Wibberley *et al* (Journal of Medical Genetics, 1977, 14, 339); M R Moore *et al* (The Lancet, 1977, i, 717).

7. See M R Moore in *Toxic effects of environmental lead* (The Conservation Society, London, 1979). The 1980 Glasgow study of newborn babies is also highly relevant here—it was scheduled to be reported in the Lawther document but did not become public until after its publication.

For a detailed technical critique of the Lawther Report, see the Conservation Society's 'counter-report' *Lead or health*, available for £2.50 from the Society's Pollution Working Party, 68 Dora Road, London SW19.

lead was deposited in the placenta or transferred to the foetus at an increasing rate'. Further research by Alexander, being published this year, shows that 'lead is significantly higher on the foetal side of the placenta as against the maternal side of the placenta in babies who are born with severe congenital abnormalities or are still-born. This indicates that there is storage of lead on the foetal side of the placenta which may be related to the abnormality or the stillbirth.'

Given that the working party was charged with producing a definitive analysis of the evidence on lead hazards, these omissions are, to say the least, intriguing.

Despite the fact that the evidence against lead in petrol has continued to pile up since March 1980—some, ironically, from work done by members of the Lawther working party—the group remains unconvinced.

For example, in May 1981 at a conference on *Lead and other pollutants—more city hazards?* at the North East London Polytechnic, Professor Lawther claimed of the Needleman study that 'You can drive a coach and horses through it statistically and in other ways'. In June 1981, at an occupational health symposium at Bury St Edmunds, Dr H A Waldron not only made his farting gnat remark, but also maintained that by reducing the lead content in petrol the Government had spent an 'excessive sum on a trivial biological matter'[8].

---

8. Reported in *Medical News* (25 June 1981).

The Government's response to Lawther

THE GOVERNMENT did not announce what action it would take following the Lawther Report until May 1981—14 months after it was published. A fierce interdepartmental argument had gone on between the DHSS, the DoE, the Treasury, the Department of Energy and the Department of Transport over leaded petrol. The DHSS had been 'knocked sideways' by the preliminary results of a study of lead levels in a group of Greenwich children. This was being carried out by two of the Lawther working party scientists, Dr Lansdown and Yule. Their results seemed to back up the Needleman evidence, indicating that children with raised lead levels (but still within the accepted normal level) could suffer an IQ loss of up to 7 points.

The other Departments, sympathetic to the pressures from the oil and motor industries, pushed for little or no action to reduce, let alone eliminate, lead in petrol.

Internal DHSS documents state that Professor Lawther was having second thoughts about his working party's view on the issue and presented fresh evidence to DHSS officials. The professor denies this.

On 11 May 1981, Tom King, the Minister for Local Government and Environmental Services, announced that the lead content in petrol would be reduced from the present 0.40 grams of lead per litre of petrol to 0.15 grams per litre (g/l) not later than by the end of 1985. In effect, the Government accepted that lead is a major threat to children but had decided not to eliminate that threat—merely to attempt to reduce the risk of damage.

The rest of the Government's proposals were equally restrained. No additional statutory regulations were announced. The paint code remains voluntary. A greater urgency in reducing the risk of lead in water was called for. Discussions would begin with local authority associations on making the replacement of domestic lead plumbing eligible for home improvement grants. The EEC air quality standard for lead of 2 micrograms of lead per cubic metre of air was adopted for the UK. The emphasis though was primarily on providing more information and advice about lead hazards.

In addition, the Government 'invited the Medical Research Council to commission a major study' on the effects of lead on children's intelligence. It had already asked the Food Additives and Contaminants Committee to study the implications of the use of lead solder in cans[1]. Finally, the Government endorsed the high blood-lead level of 35ug/100ml as the point at which action should be taken—although it did indicate that 30ug/100ml might be a more advisable limit[2].

Environment Minister, Tom King, declared: 'The report makes clear the need to improve our knowledge of the effects of lead in our environment, and particularly of possible effects on children's intelligence.' So while acknowledging the danger of leaded petrol to children (why else reduce the level of lead?), the Government was still not prepared publicly to accept or spell out just what those dangers are. To do so would have obliged considerably more action than it announced. It clearly wished to seem to be acting to eliminate dangers, but within the limits set by the oil and motor industry lobby. The result was to promote the idea that lead reduction was somehow better than lead elimination.

The Government claims that it is more effective to reduce the lead content of petrol than to go lead-free. Emissions of lead into the atmosphere would drop immediately 'by about two thirds'. And the DoE has produced a deceptively simple graph to make its point. Going lead-free, says the DoE, would have to be a gradual process over 25 years while cars are adapted or manufactured to run on lead-free petrol. It would be at least 2001 before the UK was lead-free. But reducing the lead level to 0.15g/l would produce benefits in terms of lower lead emissions by 1985 that would not be attained by 1995 if the lead-free path was followed.

The graph is a deception. First, it ignores the experience of other countries which have gone either lead-free or for major reduction. Both can be achieved much more quickly. Australia announced in 1981 that it would go lead-free by 1985, and some scientists believe it can be done by 1983. Sweden went from 0.40g/l to 0.15g/l within a year, not in 5 as the UK intends.

Second, it ignores the fact that cars will still be pumping out dangerous lead particles well into the 21st century if we only reduce the lead-level.

Third, particles from lower leaded petrol are smaller than high leaded petrol and more readily absorbed by human lungs. Thus the quantity would be reduced but the 'quality' of the poison enhanced. The Depart-

---

1. New regulations on the maximum permitted levels of lead in food has also come into force from April 1980—Lead in Food Regulations 1979 (SI 1254, HMSO).

2. See the debate on lead pollution in the House of Commons *Hansard* (11 May 1981, columns 483 to 491, HMSO).

EFFECTS ON LEAD EMISSIONS OF LEAD-FREE AND LOW-LEAD PETROL

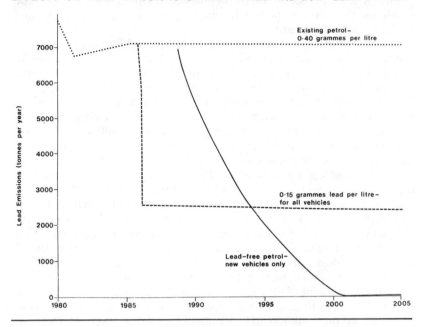

The Department of the Environment graph which purports to show why it is better to reduce the lead content of petrol to 0.15g/l rather than to go lead-free.

ment of the Environment's graph notwithstanding, reduction—of whatever size—is just not enough.

Current West German experience is confirming that going lead-free is the only effective and safe option. In 1976, the lead level in West German petrol was dropped from 0.40g/l to 0.15g/l. Research in the cities is now showing that the anticipated reductions in air lead pollution and in adults' blood lead levels are not taking place. For example, in Frankfurt air lead levels went down in proportion to petrol-lead reduction only in the immediate vicinity of busy main roads. But ambient levels—in the city air overall—fell by much less. Blood lead levels in three cities dropped by only 10 per cent, much less than expected.

One interpretation is that this shows petrol lead to be only a minor influence on blood lead levels. The other view is that in the first place it is too early for adult blood lead levels to be affected significantly by the reduction in petro lead levels, and second that low-lead petrol throws out the smaller and more easily absorbed particles.

As yet, this German cities' evidence is not definitive either way. What *is* significant is that the West German Government is negotiating with its oil industry for a further reduction in petrol lead levels.

The UK Department of Transport though has another excuse for not going lead-free. EEC regulations specify 0.15g/l as the minimum permitted level in the Community. Article 2 of EEC directive (78/611/EEC) dated 29 June 1978 states: '... a Member State may require, in respect of petrol placed upon its market, that the maximum permitted lead content be less than 0.40g/l. However, it shall not establish limits lower than 0.15g/l.'

On 11 May, the then Transport Secretary, Norman Fowler, said: 'Some people will be disappointed that we have not now committed ourselves to seeking the complete elimination of lead from petrol in the longer term. We have not done so because this is an issue which cannot be decided by the UK on its own.'

However, the DoE didn't agree. Environment Minister, Tom King, said the same day: '... although the EEC directive fixes a minimum level in the Community there is nothing to prevent the use of a lower level in this country.' The Departments subsequently deny there is any disagreement. They 'reconcile' the two statements by saying that Mr King was referring to the fact that while the directive prevents Governments from implementing a level under 0.15, it does not prevent the oil companies from producing and selling petrol under that level—should they wish to do so.

None the less, the restrictions in the EEC regulations are now seen as a temporary stumbling block for going leadfree—because they are being used as an excuse by government for *not* banning lead in petrol (see House of Commons *Hansard* 9 February 1982, cols 854/5). Some of the UK Members of the European Parliament are attempting to alter the EEC directive on lead in petrol to insist that all cars marketed in the Community should from 1 January 1985 be manufactured to take lead-free petrol and be required to run on leadfree petrol.

Perhaps the most devastating indictment both of the Lawther Report and of the Government's attitude to lead in petrol occurred in February this year. For it was revealed that the Chief Medical Officer at the Department of Health and Social Security, Sir Henry Yellowlees, had himself rejected the key findings of the Lawther Report on lead in petrol.

He had stated his position in a letter dated 6 March 1981 to Sir James Hamilton, the Permanent Secretary at the Department of Education and Science. That letter was acquired by CLEAR—the Campaign for Lead-free Air—and leaked to *The Times* on 8 February 1982. Yellowlees warned Hamilton of the 'potentially important educational implications' of the lead in petrol issue. He went on:

I must now make my own position clear. A year ago when the Lawther Report was published there was a degree of uncertainty, but since then further evidence has accrued which though not in itself wholly conclusive, nevertheless strongly supports the view that:
(a) Even at low blood levels there is a negative correlation between blood lead

levels and IQ of which the simplest explanation is that the lead produces these effects.

(b) Lead in petrol is a major contributor to blood lead acting through the food-chain as well as by inhalation[3]. Further research is being mounted but we are dealing here with the biological sciences where truly conclusive evidence may be unobtainable and it is therefore doubtful whether there is anything to be gained by deferring a decision until the results of further research become available.

There is a strong likelihood that lead in petrol is permanently reducing the IQ of many of our children. Although the reduction amounts to only a few percentage points, some hundreds of thousands of children are affected and as Chief Medical Officer I have advised my Secretary of State that action should now be taken to reduce markedly the lead content of petrol in use in the United Kingdom.

The risk to children is now shown to be too great for me to take any other course and I am therefore conveying this advice to you as Permanent Secretary in DES and I am copying the letter to the Permanent Secretaries at the Home Office and the Department of the Environment being the other Government Departments to which I owe responsibility.

You will know that several other major industrial nations faced with similar problems have opted for lead-free petrol or for petrol with a very low lead level despite the substantial costs and the energy penalties so incurred.

I regard this as a very serious issue on which I should give you my opinion as Chief Medical Officer.

Why, then, did Ministers and civil servants ignore the advice of the country's Chief Medical Officer? And why was his advice suppressed?

Not surprisingly, Sir Henry closed ranks and loyally defended the actions of his colleagues and employers. In a letter to *The Times* (13 February 1982) he wrote: 'It is erroneous to infer that my advice in any way negated or contradicted that of Professor Lawther's working party on lead and health. The contrary is the case.' He concluded by saying that the government *did* act on his advice by reducing the level of lead in petrol to 0.15g/l.

---

3. Sir Henry Yellowlees quoted fresh evidence from Italy which 'indicates that petrol lead may contribute on average about 27 per cent of total blood lead in adults, from all sources, (including food) and about 40 per cent of total blood lead in children'. He concluded: 'So the pieces in the jigsaw gradually fit together and become complete.'

The evidence against lead in petrol

ONE MAJOR FLAW of the Lawther Report is that it had scant respect for the research studies that, since the sixties, have been building up the case for taking lead out of petrol—most notably the Needleman study of over 2,000 New York children between 1975 and 1978. Here is a rundown of some of those key studies.

Rabinowitz (1972) in California found that crops of lettuce and oats were substantially polluted by leaded petrol fumes. A survey of Southern California showed that car exhaust lead travelled between 50 and 100 kilometres. The research concluded: 'If lead were removed from gasoline, there would be an immediate decrease of about 80 per cent in the lead content of crops with a subsequent decrease in human exposure.'
(See *Chemosphere* no. 4, pages 175-180, 1972, Pergamon Press)

Hrdina and Winneke (1978) in West Germany in a pilot study confirmed, if cautiously, a link between lead and children's level of ability. High-leaded children were more impaired in manual and visual co-ordination, intellectual speed and ability than low-leaded children. The more reliable method of taking tooth rather than blood samples was used. The results parallel Needleman's, and have been confirmed in more recent (1981) studies by this group.
(Paper for German Association of Hygiene and Microbiology, Mainz, October 1978; see *Toxic effects of environmental lead,* Conservation Society, May 1979)

Tjell, Hovmand and Mosbaek (1979) in Denmark found that the 'deposition of atmospheric lead on the plant surface was responsible for between 90 and 99 per cent of total lead content in the grass' in rural areas of the country.
(See *Nature* 2 August 1979, vol 280, pages 425-6)

Garnys, Freeman and Smythe (1979) in Sydney found significant differences in lead levels between urban and rural children explicable only by

airborne lead. There were also links between high-lead levels and children's performance and behaviour in school. They found high blood lead levels in children with anti-social and delinquent tendencies.
(See *Lead burdens of Sydney schoolchildren,* University of New South Wales)

Billick (1979) in New York analysed the blood lead levels of over 178,000 children during a period when leadfree petrol was being introduced (1970-77). The study found a 'highly significant' association between the airborne lead levels and the children's lead levels, and between the amount of lead present in the petrol sold and the children's lead levels. In effect, the children's lead levels rose and fell in relation to the amount of petrol lead around.

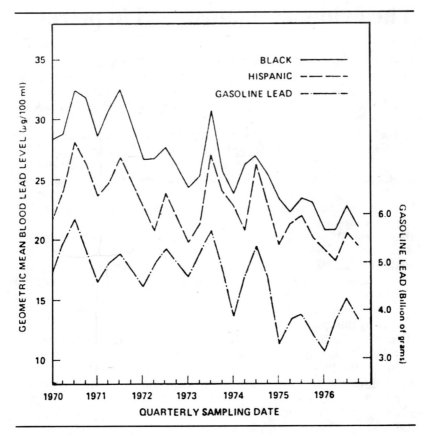

The Billick study (1) *Blood lead levels in New York children go up and down according to the rise and fall in the amount of leaded petrol sold in the city over a seven year period.*

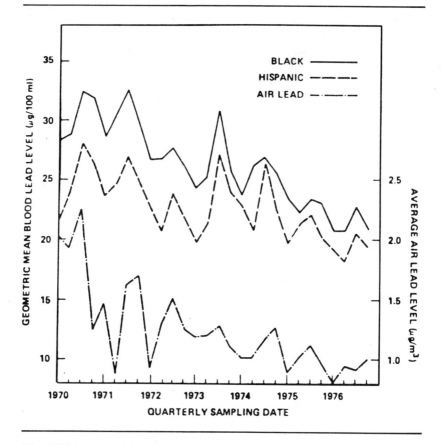

The Billick study (2) *The pattern is repeated in the comparison between the children's blood lead levels and the city's airborne lead levels over the same period. (In each case, the blood lead levels of white children were similar to those of the Hispanic children.)*

(See graphs; from report to the Department of Housing & Urban Development, Washington DC, 1979)

Needleman (1979) in Boston, USA, used the most detailed set of tests so far to show that from a group of over 2,000 children, those with elevated lead levels performed less well on a range of behaviour characteristics and abilities than those with low lead levels. Tooth (dentine) samples were used to check lead levels; teachers rated the performance and behaviour of children in school; parents completed a detailed questionnaire to account for 39 non-lead variables; a battery of neurobehavioural assessment tests were given measuring intelligence, academic achievement,

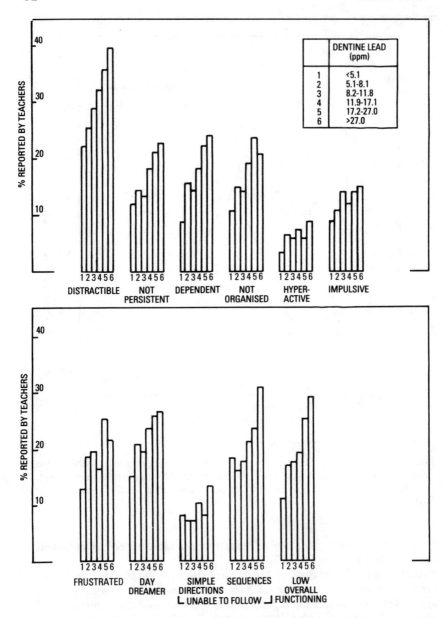

The Needleman study *2,146 New England children were studied across a range of classroom behaviour. Those with the highest lead levels (bar 6) came out worst on 9 out of 11 behaviour ratings. Overall, children's performance progressively worsened as their lead levels increased.*

auditory and language processing, visual motor coordination and attentional performance.

The researchers allowed for such 'variables' as child's physical condition, past medical history, mother's age at child's birth, family size, parental IQ and socio-economic status. The condition of pica in a child was also taken into account.

On behaviour, high-leaded children came out worse in ten out of 11 areas. The general trend was established that the higher the lead level the poorer the behaviour (see chart). One conclusion drawn from this part of the study was that 'lead may increase the risk of undesirable behaviour in the classroom at doses considerably below those found in our group with high lead levels'.

On IQ, the study found that 'the percentage of high lead children with deficient (below 75) IQ scores is three times that in the low lead group'. While no low lead children had verbal IQ scores below 72, 4.8 per cent of high lead children had scores below 66. At the upper end of the distribution, no high lead child had an IQ score greater than 125, while 4 per cent of low lead children did. Needleman concluded:

> The impaired function of children with high lead levels, demonstrated in the neuropsychological laboratory, mirrored by disordered classroom behaviour, appears to be an early adverse effect of exposure to lead. Permissible exposure levels of lead for children deserve re-examination in the light of these data. (March 1979)

Needleman and his colleagues identified four major defects in previous lead studies, and took account of them in their own research study. These were: (1) Inadequate indicators of lead exposure—blood samples were commonly used; Needleman used the more reliable tooth samples. (2) Insensitive measures of performance—group tests or mass screening exams cannot detect subtle changes. (3) Inadequate attention to non-lead variables which can also affect development in children, such as socio-economic status, parental rearing style, parental intelligence, medical history. (4) Selection bias—the way people are selected to be the subjects of a survey can upset or bias the results; Needleman points out: 'Studies that select their subjects from health clinics, schools for the retarded or psychiatric clinics may not be representative of the population in general. Similarly, families who fear that their child has a deficit may respond to a study invitation in a systematically biased fashion, and either seek or avoid participation, depending on how the study is perceived.'

(See *Deficits in psychologic and classroom performance of children with elevated dentine lead levels* in The New England Journal of Medicine, 29 March 1979, vol 300, no 13)

Rutter (1980) reviewed the evidence thus far on raised lead levels and impaired cognitive/behavioural functioning. On the Needleman study, he concluded that it

> provides the most impressive evidence to date on the possible damaging effects

of raised lead levels in the range usually previously considered harmless, and which are found in some 20 per cent of children in the general population. There are a number of important questions and reservations about the study and the inferences to be drawn from it, but none of these are sufficient to invalidate the findings.

On the evidence as a whole, Dr Michael Rutter concluded:

> The cognitive deficits which have been found have usually been of the order of 3 to 5 points, and it has been argued that a 5-point difference is so trivial in its effects that it can be safely ignored. That is a totally fallacious argument... a drop of 5 points in mean IQ... for any population must necessarily result in more than a two-fold increase in the percentage of individuals with an IQ below 70 ie. a *doubling* of the number of mentally retarded children!

Dr Rutter was a member of the Lawther working party. He was the only one to discuss the Needleman study *with* Dr Needleman. The Lawther Report said of the Needleman study:

> Together these studies (Needleman et al, 1979; Hrdina and Winneke, 1978) provide some evidence of an association between raised tooth dentine lead levels and a slight lowering of measured intelligence. There are a number of reservations about these studies and the inferences to be drawn from them which in our view weakens their conclusions. (para 159, page 68)

Later, the Report states (incorrectly):

> Needleman et al (1979) report near-linear relationships between tooth lead level and distractibility, lack of persistence, impulsivity and daydreaming. Unfortunately the rating scale items were not standardised and social and other factors were not taken into account.
>
> In summary it can be stated that up to the present no study has satisfactorily demonstrated a relationship between increasing body lead burden and either educational attainment or hyperactivity.
> (paras 167-8, page 72)

The Lawther working party did not have, nor did they seek access to the full details of the Needleman study, which showed that Needleman and his colleagues had accounted for those factors while the Lawther group claimed they had not.

For a time, a minority report was being considered by a few members of the Lawther working party disagreeing with the official line on lead in petrol and on the relationship between lead levels and effects on behaviour. In the end, nothing came of it—the Rutter paper seems the nearest thing to a minority report.

(See *Raised lead levels and impaired cognitive/behavioural functioning: a review of the evidence;* Supplement to Developmental Medicine and Child Neurology, vol 22 no 1, March 1980)

Yule and Lansdown (1981) carried out a pilot study of 166 Greenwich children on the relationship between blood lead levels and intelligence and attainment. The study found blood lead levels ranging between 7 and

33ug/100ml (within the 'normal' range of lead levels where lead is, officially, not supposed to have any detrimental effects). 'Significant associations' were recorded between these levels and attainment scores on tests of reading, spelling and intelligence—but not of mathematics.

The children were divided into those with a blood-lead level of 12ug/100ml and below, and those of 13ug/100ml and above. The 'high lead' group had an average full scale IQ deficit of *7 points* compared with the 'low lead' group.

Drs Yule and Lansdown, both members of the Lawther working party, are extremely cautious about their results, which appear to support the Needleman evidence. Indeed, they suggest an even greater damaging link between lead and intelligence for Needleman found a 5 point IQ deficit. They conclude:

> Before asserting that the associations seen in the present study offer any support for the notion that there is a relationship between blood lead concentrations within the normal range and functioning at school, it will be necessary to do further work, paying greater attention to social factors.

That work is now underway.

(See *The relationship between blood lead concentrations, intelligence and attainment in a school population: a pilot study* in Developmental Medicine and Child Neurology, October 1981, pages 567-76)

Taking action

FOUR MAIN options are available for doing something about the hazard of leaded petrol:
1 Fitting lead filters to cars to 'trap' the lead and prevent it from getting into the air.
2 Using alternative fuels for motor vehicles.
3 Reducing the level of lead added to petrol.
4 Switching to leadfree petrol.

Lead filters

There is considerable support for lead filters within the oil and motor industries. Associated Octel has carried out detailed tests on filters with, it claims, good results. The Fellowship of Engineering also favours filters as a response to the leaded petrol problem that it considers to be cheap, quick to implement and effective:

> The lead filter option could be introduced more quickly... and could produce reductions of up to 50% in lead emission with virtually no energy penalty.

However, they conclude, in a report[1] on lead in the environment:

> In view of the findings of the Lawther Committee... we suggest that careful consideration should be given to the costs in terms of economics and energy, and the benefits in terms of improved health and lessened risks, before further restrictive legislation is introduced. The question should be asked as to whether our limited finances could not be spent in some other more productive or beneficial way.

A revised version of the report was issued in August 1981 following the

---

1. *Reduction of lead in the environment—energy, technology and costs* (Fellowship of Engineering, December 1980).

Government's response to the Lawther report. An additional sentence was included in the report's final paragraph quoted above. This read: 'Unless the medical evidence becomes incontrovertible, there appears to be very little justification to go to the complete elimination of lead.'

Other agencies and countries are less enthusiastic about lead filters. Several countries have, after tests, rejected them as inefficient (failing to trap a sufficient amount of lead) and dangerous (creating a new problem of disposal after use). Some tests have shown that lead filters tend only to trap the large particles of lead but allow the small, and more dangerous, ones to escape.

Alternative fuels

Another option is for vehicles to use a fuel other than petrol. Diesel fuel is unleaded, produces less pollution and is cheaper than petrol. However, diesel cars do cost more to buy and some have a poorer performance than their petrol-powered equivalents. In the UK, diesel cars comprise only 0.6 per cent of new car sales.

A cheaper and more practical alternative is a liquefied petroleum gas (LPG) fuel—in effect, propane and butane gas. LPG's advantages are that it is substantially cheaper than petrol (up to two-thirds cheaper), does not significantly affect performance, reduces engine wear and maintenance costs. As with leadfree petrol, cars require either hardened exhaust valves or a special cylinder head to prevent the engine's valve seats from burning out—conversion cost is currently reckoned at between £75 and £100.

LPG is seen as a major alternative to leaded petrol by many other European countries. For example, 10 per cent of petrol-engine vehicles in Italy and Holland run on LPG.

In 1980, the West German Government began secret talks with its oil industry to negotiate a further reduction in its petrol lead level, currently 0.15g/l: in the face of the industry's objections and warnings of higher costs, it has decided to invest in an LPG conversion programme as an alternative.

Converting half a million of West Germany's 24 million vehicles would, it is claimed by the oil and motor industries, reduce the total amount of lead discharged into the air to the level required. The plan, supported by tax incentives, is to convert 100,000 vehicles a year for 5 years. The major petrol companies are setting up refuelling points at filling stations.

Such a programme is feasible for the UK. By 1985, Britain will have an extra 5 million tons of LPG available from the North Sea oilfields. Half a million vehicles require 750,000 to 1 million tons of LPG annually. So the fuel is there. Ford has just produced an LPG version of its Transit van. Test programmes are underway at BL and Vauxhall, Volkswagen and

Talbot. Special cylinder heads are already available for Ford vehicles[2].

A capital investment programme would be needed to set up the necessary infrastructure for vehicle conversion and fuel distribution. So far, only 40,000 vehicles in the UK use LPG—mainly local authority owned vehicles. In London, there are only 50 LPG refuelling points.

Taking the lead out

The main argument has focused on whether to reduce the amount of lead in petrol—and if so by how much—or to go leadfree. The oil, and motor industries have successfully put pressure on Government ministers and civil servants over many years to see things their way.

In 1978, Denis Howell, then a minister at the DoE, admitted that his advisers were giving him incomplete advice on the health hazards of lead. In January 1979, Tory MP for Epsom, Archie Hamilton, said in the Commons:

> I have received the overwhelming impression from the oil companies that not only do they not want to make an expensive reduction in petrol lead levels, but they are putting pressure on the Government to persuade them to do nothing. A pressure, alas, to which this Government seems only too willing to succumb.

The industries have always been deeply influential in numerous government-sponsored studies to assess the effects of lead in petrol[3]. For example, in July 1979 a feasibility study[4] by the Department of Transport (assisted by oil company and motor trade representatives) set out five options for limiting lead in petrol. The cost of the options—worked out by the oil companies—ranged from £70 million (for fitting lead filters in cars) to £200 million (for producing leadfree and better refined petrol). All the options would, claimed the report, mean extra expense for the consumer and increased consumption of oil. The report failed to consider, or to cost, the benefits—health, environmental and financial—that could accrue from lower leaded or leadfree petrol.

In February 1982, a report commissioned by CLEAR (the Campaign for Lead-free Air) from management consultants Coopers and Lybrand criticised the 1979 feasibility study for overlooking the most practical way to go leadfree. This was to reduce the lead level in petrol to 0.15g/l and, at the same time, to require all new cars to run on leadfree petrol. Such a

---

2. In general terms engines with cast iron cylinder heads subject to high speed, full load operation will experience high wear rate of the exhaust valve seat area. However, if a hardened valve seat insert is fitted, this problem is cured. Engines fitted with aluminium cylinder heads do have a valve seat insert fitted as standard and experience indicates the hardness value of these inserts is adequate for LPG operation. Examples of such engines are in the Volvo 244, Rover and Princess ranges, and most Japanese cars.

3. See also the Harwell research studies, page 30.

4. *Lead in petrol:* an assessment of the feasibility and costs of further action to limit lead emissions from vehicles (Dept of Transport/Petroleum Industry Advisory Committee/Society of Motor Trade Manufacturers).

package would have achieved the fastest reduction of lead emissions from cars, the gradual introduction of leadfree petrol, and an end to uncertainty for the oil and motor industries. (See *The polluting effects of lead in petrol* by Coopers and Lybrand, and CLEAR Newsletter for May 1982.)

In addition, an analysis carried out by Friends of the Earth estimates that going leadfree would save almost 400,000 tonnes of oil a year. This contradicts government estimates that leadfree petrol would put up the UK's oil consumption by one per cent. The FoE report *Lead in petrol: an energy analysis* by Brian Price (February 1982) says that savings would be achieved through improved mileage per gallon and longer engine and exhaust wear for cars run on leadfree petrol. Further, energy costs from the manufacture and transport of the lead additives would be saved.

Leadfree petrol is not only better for humans, it is better for cars too—providing a longer life for exhausts and engines. For along with the lead have to be added lead scavengers in order to slow down the build up of damaging lead deposit in the car engine. Such scavengers work by generating hydrochloric acid in the combustion chamber and are eventually expelled through the car exhaust. The hydrochloric acid gradually corrodes the iron and steel used in the car engine and also attacks the car's lubricating oil. In addition, the financial and energy costs of producing lead additives would be saved; the dangers of transporting highly poisonous chemicals for additive production across the country would be avoided; the risk to wild life in the land and water around the Associated Octel lead-additive production site would end.

Such elements are rarely put into the lead equation by Government—and certainly not by industry. In short, successive Governments have followed where the oil and motor industries have wanted them to go.

Both the Government and the UK oil industry claim that leadfree petrol cannot be produced in sufficient quantity until 1990 at the earliest. Merely reducing the lead level from the present 0.40 to 0.15 grams per litre (g/l) will take up to four years. Yet the oil industry was planning to produce leadfree petrol during 1979 in a matter of months to combat the effects of industrial disputes. And as early as 1971, Shell and BP had said that they could provide leadfree petrol 'as and when required'[5]. Burmah was planning to introduce it as a technically superior fuel, but could not secure the necessary co-operation from the rest of the oil industry.

During the 78/9 winter, lead additives for petrol could not be delivered to the refineries from the Associated Octel plant at Ellesmere Port, Britain's sole producer of lead additives. To conserve stocks already held at the refineries, the level of lead in the petrol supplied to filling stations was severely reduced, often below the 0.15g/l level. A small amount of leadfree petrol was also produced by Esso—and other companies were preparing to go leadfree when their lead stocks ran out.

The Amoco oil company has stated that it is considering the possibility

5. *Processing* magazine, July 1981.

of marketing leadfree petrol in the UK—and that had government required it, Amoco could have produced leadfree fuel ten years ago. (Report in *The Sunday Times*, 14 February 1982).

Yet oil companies and the British Government still argue that the changeover process is too complex, too expensive, and that cars currently in production could not cope with the 'new' petrol produced. At Texaco, an internal policy memo, to alert staff to the official public line on lead reduction, prepared a week after the Government's May 1981 announcement stated:

> Texaco's present manufacturing facilities, even after the new Catalytic Cracker at Pembroke is brought into operation in 1982 do not have the capability to produce petrol containing 0.15g/litre at current octane levels in the volume required for Texaco's sales in the UK. Additional investment in new processing equipment will be required either in the UK or elsewhere in Europe.
>
> In view of the new processing facilities required it is unlikely that Texaco would be prepared to market the reduced lead petrol in advance of the Government mandated date which was in fact designed to permit adequate time for the oil industry to adjust production to the new lead level.

Other countries have reduced lead levels in petrol in a much shorter time than the British Government claims is needed. In Sweden, the cooperatively-run OK Oil Company switched to a lead level of 0.15g/l within a year of deciding to do so. Scientists in Australia, which expects to go leadfree in 1985, maintain the change can be made by 1983.

The experience of other countries also challenges the British claim that leadfree petrol will be considerably more expensive to produce—and therefore to sell. The British Government says 0.15g/l leaded petrol will cost the motorist 4p a gallon extra—at 1981 prices. Leadfree petrol would be more. But in Sweden the same lead grade petrol cost an extra 1.5p a gallon more for 4-star, and 0.75p for 2-star. In West Germany, there was no increase in the price of petrol at that lead grade.

Refining costs in West Germany were also well below the estimated figures produced by the British Government. Low-leaded and leadfree petrol has to be refined to a higher standard, and requires more crude oil in its manufacture—up to ½ million tonnes a year for leadfree petrol. For without the lead, the octane rating drops and this has to be maintained in other, more expensive, ways. The Transport Ministry of the West German Government says of the investment costs for switching to 0.15g/l leaded petrol:

> The overall investment of all 25 refineries—Dm227.5 million—is nowhere near the total of Dm1,000 million predicted and published by the oil industry.

Eighty per cent of UK cars need high-octane 4-star petrol and, allegedly, cannot run on petrol with a lead level under 0.15g/l without engine modifications. But the octane rating in the 1979 'emergency' petrol was reduced by half an octane—and the lead level dipped below the 0.15g/l mark with no detrimental effects.

To run permanently on leadfree petrol, the majority of cars sold in Britain do need engine modification. Again both the extent and the cost of such modifications have been exaggerated by government and industry. But this the nub of the technical argument over lead in petrol.

The main problem is that lead acts as a lubricant. No lead means more engine wear. The solution is to harden the valve seats to prevent them burning out. Once this is done, there is even less engine wear and better fuel economy using leadfree petrol.

According to British Leyland, existing car ranges such as Rover and Princess have hardened cylinder heads (made of aluminium) enabling them to run up to 30,000 miles on leadfree petrol. Other BL makes, such as the Metro, have a not-so-tough cast-iron head—but they can still run up to 5,000 miles on low-octane unleaded fuel. Ford has launched a version of its Transit van which can run on leadfree petrol. The extra cost is £75.

The cost of fitting hardened valves to a car already on the road has been estimated at about £100 (including VAT) for a one-off operation, reducing to £75 if there was substantial demand for the service. Some British made cars are produced to take leadfree petrol for export; Japanese cars imported to Britain are altered to take leaded petrol.

Another option, considered even more feasible than L.P.G fuel, is to replace lead as an octane improver in petrol. One attractive octane-booster being investigated is Methyl Tertiary Butyl Ether (MTBE). It is derived from coal and natural gas, and made from two chemicals, methanol and isobutylene. A Scottish-based chemical processing consortium, Highland Hydrocarbons, is planning to produce MTBE eventually to supply up to half the amount of octane boosters needed for the UK market. (See "*Some alternative to lead in petrol*" by Michael Pettman, CALIP, March 1982.)

In America, oil companies and the car industry are more willing to admit and to promote the advantages of leadfree petrol and of alternative forms of motor fuel. In 1972, the Society of Automotive Engineers published the results of a 5-year survey[6] on the difference in maintenance costs for cars operated by leadfree as opposed to leaded premium petrol. The survey concluded:

> Leadfree gasolines typically cost slightly more than leaded gasolines, and a frequently raised question concerns why a customer should pay this higher price. Our work has shown that the steady use of lead-free gasoline ensures significant savings with maintenance costs. Eliminating the lead antiknock compounds from the gasoline unquestionably reduces or postpones the need for exhaust system repairs, spark plug replacements, carburetor servicing, and other gasoline-related maintenance. Moreover, no adverse side effects such as valve seat wear have been observed.

The level of maintenance costs saved over the lifetime of an average car more than offsets the extra cost of leadfree gasoline at the pumps.

6. *Saving maintenance dollars with lead-free gasoline* by D S Gray and A G Azhari of the American Oil Company (Society of Automotive Engineers Congress, January 1972).

What next?

IN A REPORT prepared by the American Committee on Lead in the
Human Environment for the National Academy of Sciences in 1980,
Clair Patterson writes:

> Extrapolating from present data, there is some basis for believing that it will be
> shown in the future that significant irreversible deleterious effects to the central
> nervous systems of some ten thousand inner-city babies are being caused each
> year in the United States by exposures to industrial lead.
>
> Extrapolating from present information, it also seems probable, from the
> viewpoint of cellular biochemistry, that it will be shown in the future that
> average American adults experience a variety of significant physiological and
> intellectual dysfunctions caused by long-term chronic lead insult to their bodies
> and minds which results from excess exposures to industrial lead that are five
> hundred-fold above natural levels of lead exposure, and that such dysfunctions
> on this massive scale may have significantly influenced the course of American
> history.

Patterson believes that 'in the near future it probably will be shown that
the older urban areas of the United States have been rendered more or
less uninhabitable by the millions of tons of poisonous industrial lead
residues that have accumulated in cities during the past century'.

The Committee comprised the Environmental Studies Board, the
Commission on Natural Resources, and the National Research Council.

The Committee's report was requested by the US Department of
Housing and Urban Development. It wanted to know whether lead from
house paints or lead from petrol had the greater influence on inner-city
babies. Patterson and his colleagues realised that 'a report issued according to engineering perspectives and traditions of the past would not
provide specific guidance that would enable HUD or the Congress to
significantly reduce within a short time, by regulatory action or statute,
lead poisoning among inner-city babies.' In effect, the costs allegedly

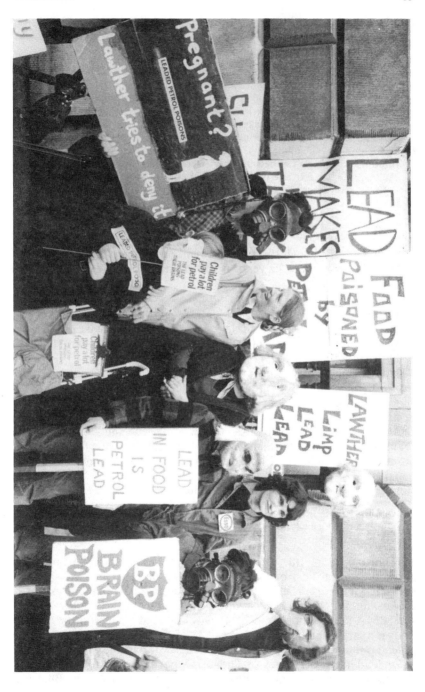

involved and the attitudes of the relevant professions would militate against action being taken: the arguments put up in Britain. Patterson succinctly stated the dilemma:

> My view is that sufficient information is available to indicate that steps should be initiated now to reduce and eventually halt the mining and smelting of lead and the manufacture of leaded products within the shortest possible time, that the manufacturing of some leaded products be halted forthwith, and that immediate steps should be taken to clean up existing lead residues and render them nonhazardous. Traditional engineering views avoid this issue. Instead, such views that the mining and smelting of lead and the dispersal of manufactured lead products can be safely carried out under proper controls, and that the real problem is to find out exactly where the lead is going and exactly which types of exposures are harmful, so that the proper type of controls can be instituted.

It is worth remembering that the United States has more stringent controls than Britain.

In July 1981, Dr Herbert Needleman, speaking at a Swedish symposium on his previous six years' work on lead levels, said:

> ... the case seems strong indeed that lead at low dose is an important and widely distributed neurotoxin. Unlike many neuropsychiatric diseases, little remains to be discovered about lead poisoning. The etiology, some of the biochemical toxicology, and the necessary steps to eliminate the problem are clearly spelled out. The larger challenges with lead lie in finding the will and the means to remove it from the human environment.

UK Government departments, satisfied that the decision merely to reduce the lead in petrol in four years' time is enough, refuse to contemplate further discussion—let alone action. Last July, the Inner London Education Authority passed a resolution urging the complete removal of lead from petrol. It also requested a meeting with the Department of Transport, along with teacher and parent groups, to discuss their concern for inner city children. The Department refused to meet them and remains unconvinced that lead in petrol damages children. The Transport Department's Permanent Secretary replied to ILEA:

> There is I think little to add at this stage, as far as evidence or arguments are concerned, which would justify a meeting between us. The issues have already been very well aired.

In February 1982, the British Medical Association (BMA) publicly became more critical of lead in petrol and declared it is considering pressing for more cuts in the amount of lead in the environment. A BMA spokesman stated on 9 February: 'On the basis of past scientific evidence the (BMA's) Board of Science believes that lead taken into the human body is a serious public health hazard. The Board believes that all sources of lead pollution should be eliminated wherever possible.'

On lead in petrol, Professor Thomas Oppe, a member of the Board of Science and a member of the Lawther working party said: 'The Board...

is convinced that low level exposure to lead can be a cause of brain damage. Every effort should be made to reduce lead levels in the environment.'

The argument over lead in petrol centres on the two issues of health and the technical feasibility of producing leadfree petrol and cars that run on it. If leadfree petrol *is* on the way, say the oil companies in private, then they could readily and would prefer to produce leadfree petrol now with a low octane 2-star rating. That is less expensive than producing leadfree, high octane 4-star petrol. But that shifts the initial financial burden to the motor industry which would have to do some retooling and rejig most car engine designs to run on low rather than high octane fuel. So the motor industry wants either low-lead petrol or unleaded but high octane fuel. Thus far the Government has sided more with the motor than the oil industry, fearing for example that going leadfree means British Leyland costs increase or sales drop. For the Japanese car industry is much better placed to cope with leadfree fuel. The most practical way forward, so far rejected by the UK, is to allow existing cars to run on leaded fuel at 0.15g/l but insist that all new cars run on leadfree petrol.

As for the health issue, there is now more than enough hardcore evidence to show lead's harmful effects on children. More evidence, based on further surveys in the UK, is due over the next two to three years. What is to be done if those experts who have the ear of Government decide once again that *they* don't find the evidence convincing? Or if Government ministers and civil servants find the vested interests of industry more to their liking than the wellbeing of children?

One politician, Lord Avebury the president of the Conservation Society, put it this way:

> Can we afford to take the risk that large numbers of children and pregnant mothers will have been exposed to concentrations of lead which the scientists finally agree are enough to cause behavioural or mental disorders and educational under-achievement?
>
> This is a political question which cannot be left to the scientists alone. The scientists advise, and they differ in their opinions. Ultimately, it is for each one of us to form a judgement on the evidence presented, as to what degree of protection is needed. If we are forced to the conclusion that the health of future generations may be undermined, then it will be through the political process that remedies have to be sought. Whether or not there is a high enough level of public concern to prompt Government action, nobody... can say he or she was not warned, in the clearest terms, of an environmental disaster we may now be creating for our children. (*Lead or health*, Conservation Society, November 1980).

Campaigning against lead

THE MAIN pressure group on lead has long been the Campaign Against Lead in Petrol (CALIP) based at 68 Dora Road, London SW19 7HH (01-946 7542). It was formed out of the Conservation Society's Pollution Working Party. A linked group is Parents Against Lead (PAL) operating from 17 Holland Park Gardens, London W14 (01-603 5778). In addition, local anti-lead campaigns are organised by Friends of the Earth groups and some community health councils.

In January 1982, eight environmental and community organisations united behind a new major campaign for lead-free petrol. CLEAR—the Campaign for Lead-free Air—is supported by CALIP, the Conservation Society, Friends of the Earth, Transport 2000, the Association of Community Health Councils for England and Wales, the Advisory Centre for Education, the Association of Neighbourhood Councils, and the Health Visitors Association. (All these groups continue to campaign separately against lead as well as under the CLEAR banner.)

CLEAR is based at 2 Northdown Street, London N1 9BG (01-278 9686). This is also the base for the CLEAR Charitable Trust which will undertake research and publication on the lead issue. CLEAR has the following objectives:

1 To urge that the fixed limit of 0.15 grams per litre for lead in petrol be introduced earlier than the official date of 1985 and be for *existing cars* only.

2 To demand that as soon as possible, and in any event by early 1985, all *new cars* sold on the UK market be required to run on lead-free petrol, and that all petrol stations be required to have lead-free petrol available for sale to the public.

3 To urge that taxation on the sale of petrol should be imposed to create a price advantage to motorists purchasing lead-free petrol.

4 To maintain surveillance on the use of lead generally and to encourage

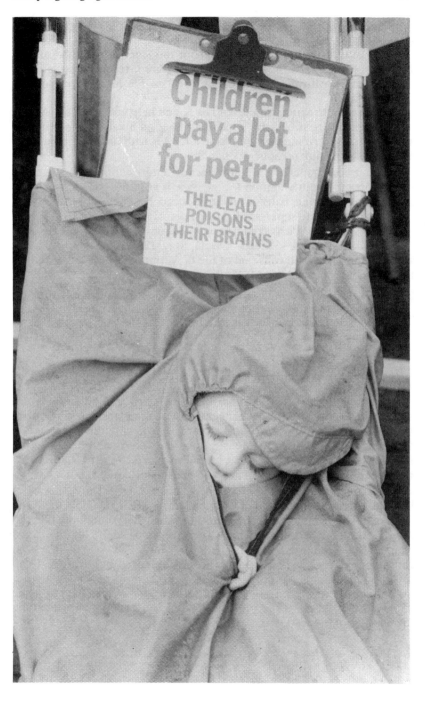

enforcement of any measures necessary to reduce lead pollution wherever it occurs.

Parents and teachers concerned about the level of pollution around their schools can raise the issue through the parent-teacher association or the school's governing body—or go direct to the local environmental health office.

Detailed information on the lead issue and help with campaigning are available both from CALIP, which publishes an invaluable information bulletin *CALIP Newsletter,* and from CLEAR with its developing information bureau and introductory handbook.

Trade union branches have now become interested in the issue and a useful forum to gain attention for the issue is at trades council meetings. In Australia, 'green bans' were introduced by Shell employees who refused to distribute super-grade leaded petrol.

The 1981 Labour Party conference voted for the next Labour Government to ban the use of lead. On 11 May 1981, Opposition Energy spokesman, Denis Howell, said of the Government's decision to reduce the lead content of petrol to 0.15g/l:

> We believe that this is the wrong decision, given the two options before the Government of either reducing the maximum to 0.15 grams per litre or going for lead-free petrol immediately. We believe that the latter decision should have been taken now... The Opposition will certainly go for lead-free petrol. (*Hansard,* 11 May 1981, col 484).

CLEAR has also acquired promises of support from Liberal and Social Democratic leaders.

Local campaigns often link the general issue of lead pollution with a specific local concern—a school near a busy road or lead smelting works, the building of a new car park or garage near children's play areas. Groups have organised demonstrations and picketed oil and motor company offices. The lead issue, especially when it concerns children, has been readily taken up by local newspapers and local radio stations.

Many organisations, well-intentioned in their own field, are unaware of the lead threat to children. For example, during 1981 the Help the Aged campaign ran a nationwide treasure-hunt for primary school children. Among the objects to be collected were pieces of lead. Help the Aged claimed that 'lead' was a printing error for 'bead'. They said there was no cause for concern as 'only one child in a hundred had collected and returned lead items'. Some 200,000 treasure-hunt forms had been sent out, which therefore put—according to Help the Aged's figure—some 2,000 children at risk. The organisation has subsequently reprinted the forms without the lead item.

What a group can do

Several schools in lead-risk areas have set up their own anti-lead group to work for better precautions for the children and to lobby for local action against lead. Such groups can also be established on a community-wide basis bringing in a range of interests for whom lead is a threat.

Information

Build up a lead library for your group—gather together as much relevant material (reports, research results, articles and so on) about lead—local, national, international. Remember you are up against the oil companies, the motor industry and the Government. You need to get your facts right, even if they don't. You also need to let other people know the facts. A local anti-lead bulletin, metings, leafletting, stalls at markets and fairs, demonstrations at zebra crossings at rush hour can all help to get the case across.

Lobbying

Identify key groups in the area that can help, and that need to be made aware about lead. Talk with them about the lead issue: groups of local doctors and nurses, health service and transport unions, environmental health officers and so on. Many remain sceptical about the lead issue because they rely only on 'official' advice from the medical establishment. EHOs—the guardians of local health—particularly need to be encouraged to see the dangers of lead pollution to children. Lobby local councillors and involve your MP and other prospective political candidates.

Action

Identify high-risk spots in your area. Persuade the local authority to test schools, play areas, and shopping areas by busy roads. Persuade local health services to offer lead level tests for children. Help to develop a local policy for official action against lead pollution sources.

Local city councillors can be encouraged to take up the lead issue on the three fronts of water supply, paint and petrol. High-risk traffic areas should be monitored closely for lead levels—the busiest routes don't always have the highest local readings because lead particles can travel some distance according to local conditions. There is nothing to prevent councils developing alternative fuel filling points and car conversion programmes for both these fuels and for leadfree petrol. Unleaded petrol could also be made available.

Lead and the law

DESPITE several test cases brought to force industries or councils to take action against lead hazards, none in this country has yet been successful. Relevant acts include the Public Health Act 1936 and the Control of Pollution Act 1974.

In a case brought by London parents, which ran for over two years, alleging damage to their children from leaded petrol, the defending oil companies referred the case to the Official Solicitor on the grounds that the parents were unfit to act on behalf of their children. They also claimed the case was 'vexatious, frivolous and an abuse of the courts'. The Official Solicitor backed the parents, but they eventually lost the case.

No-one has yet brought a case against a UK local authority for allowing lead hazards to exist in, for example, schools or playgrounds. One such case is currently pending in Stockholm.

Keeping the lead at bay

PARENTS and children can take some simple precautions that can help to slow the rate at which lead is absorbed. This is more important in urban rather than rural areas. Pregnant women, babies and young children should take special care.

Diet

● Fresh food is always better than canned food. Never give babies canned food meant for adults.
● Always wash or peel fresh fruit and vegetables, particularly if you know they've been grown in allotments or gardens beside busy roads.
● Liver, kidney and shellfish often have a high lead content.
● It helps if children have a balanced diet and are well fed—make sure they have a good breakfast.
● Some scientists recommend that a good anti-lead diet should include vitamin D, lots of pectin (eg. in fresh fruit) and trace elements such as calcium and phosphate.
● Don't buy unpackaged food from petrol stations.

Play

● Don't play in busy streets, car parks or near garage forecourts.
● Always wash hands after playing outside.
● Never pick up and eat sweets etc. dropped on the ground.
● Get your child's school to hose down the playground regularly.
● Don't let children chew or suck old or imported toys, especially if they are made of metal or if painted.

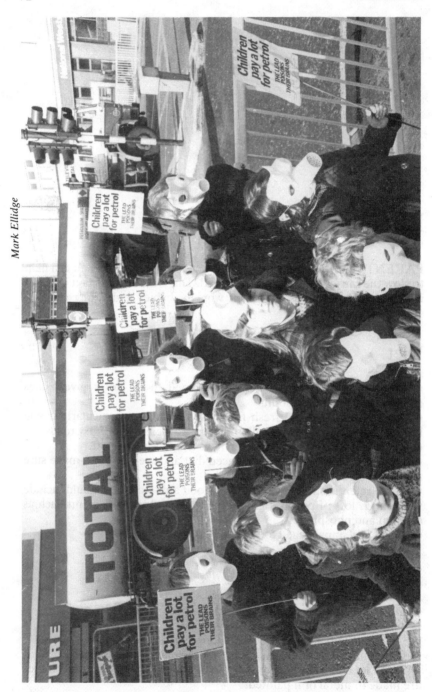

Mark Ellidge

In the street

● Don't leave babies in prams etc. near busy traffic.
● Don't stand around near traffic jams or anywhere else with car engines idling.

At home

● Keep windows facing busy streets closed.
● Keep dust off food and crockery—always wash them before use. Don't use handmade pottery for food or drink unless you are sure it is leadfree.
● Deal quickly with any peeling paint—especially if the paint is old. Never let children chew paint flakes. Keep children away when you are stripping old paint.
● Only use a water softener if you know you have no lead plumbing. Always run the tap for a minute or two before using the water.
● Don't smoke—particularly if you are pregnant. Tobacco smoke contains small amounts of poisonous metals, including lead.

For more detailed advice contact CALIP—send SAE if you write. For general information on nutrition, contact the British Nutrition Foundation, 15 Belgrave Square, London SW1 (01-235 4904). A useful book on diet is *Eating for health* (HMSO). For general information on health, contact the Health Education Council, 78 New Oxford Street, London WC1 (01-637 1881).

Where to find out more

THIS IS a selection of key reports and features providing information, analysis or opinion from a range of sources on the lead issue.

From Government
Lead and health (March 1980, the Lawther Report, DHSS, HMSO)
Lead pollution in Birmingham (1978, Pollution Paper 14, DoE, HMSO)
Lead in drinking water (1977, Pollution Paper 12, DoE, HMSO)
Lead in the environment and its significance to man (1974, Pollution Paper 2, DoE, HMSO)

From the anti-lead groups
Lead or health (November 1980, a review of contemporary lead pollution and a critique of the Lawther Report)
Toxic effects of environmental lead (May 1979, report of an international symposium on health effects of lead)
Lead pollution—health effects (April 1978, report of an international symposium)
All available from the Conservation Society Pollution Working Party, 68 Dora Road, London SW19)
Lead-free air...a legacy for our children a handbook published by CLEAR—The Campaign for Lead-free Air, 2 Northdown Street, London N1.

From the industries
Lead in petrol: an assessment of the feasibility and costs of further action to limit lead emissions from vehicles (July 1979, available from the Vehicle Standards and Engineering Division, Department of Transport,

2 Marsham Street, London SW1P 3EB)
Reduction of lead in the environment—energy, technology and cost
(August 1981, available from the Fellowship of Engineers, 2 Little Smith
Street, London SW1)

Others

The Consumers' Association produced a report on 'Water' in *Which?*
January 1980.

Articles and letters on research and opinion on lead appear frequently in
the medical journals, such as *The Lancet, British Medical Journal,* and
World Medicine. Recent examples include:

'Is low-level lead pollution dangerous?' and 'Sources of lead pollution' by
Daphne Gloag (*British Medical Journal,* 13 December 1980 and 3 January 1981).

'Lead pollution: why the government must act now' by Robin Russell-
Jones (*World Medicine,* 7 February 1981).

See also: 'Still pumping poison into our children' by Robin Russell Jones
and Derek Bryce Smith, *Futures* section of *The Guardian* (1 October 1981)

Lead pollution: causes and control by R M Harrison and D P H Laxen
(Chapman and Hall, 1981). A book that claims to adopt 'a balanced,
impartial approach' to lead pollution and methods for limiting lead
emissions.

What we use lead for

Lead has been mined and used commercially for thousands of years.
The Romans were major users of lead. In Britain, nineteenth century
industrialisation produced a massive increase in lead smelting works
and the manufacture of lead-based products. It also created a huge
pollution problem in homes and in the workplace.

Today, Britain uses around a quarter of a million tonnes of refined
lead—5.5 per cent of an annual world total of 4.4 million tonnes (1978
figures). Two thirds of that total is consumed by only eight countries—
USA, USSR, West Germany, Japan, Britain, France, China and
Italy.

Refined lead is used mainly in the electrical storage battery trade,
for cable coverings, sheeting, pipes and tubes, solders, alloys and
ammunition. One third of the lead goes into making compounds:
pigments and drying agents for paints, glazing, lubricants and stabi-
lisers for plastics.

Some 10 per cent of refined lead goes into the manufacture of
anti-knock additives for petrol—tetra-ethyl lead (TEL) and tetra-
methyl lead (TML).

Calculating lead intake from dietary and airborne lead
Diet
Daily average intake   = 113ug (MAFF, 1980)
Average absorption rate from
the gut   = 10 per cent (WHO)
Therefore: amount absorbed
from diet   = 11.3ug per day

Inhalation
Background airborne lead level
in urban areas   = 1ug/m^3
Volume of air respired per day   = 23 m^3 (US Nat Academy
                                        of Sciences)
Absorption rate from lungs range
from 48 to 64 per cent
(AERE, Harwell)   = avr 55 per cent
Amount absorbed from the air   = 55 per cent of 23ug = 12.6ug
Total absorbed from air and diet = 11.3 + 12.6 = 23.9ug
Contribution from inhaled lead   = 12.6/23.9 = 52.7 per cent
(At airborne lead level of 2ug/m^3, contribution of inhaled lead
becomes 69 per cent)

Source: Professor D Bryce-Smith, University of Reading.

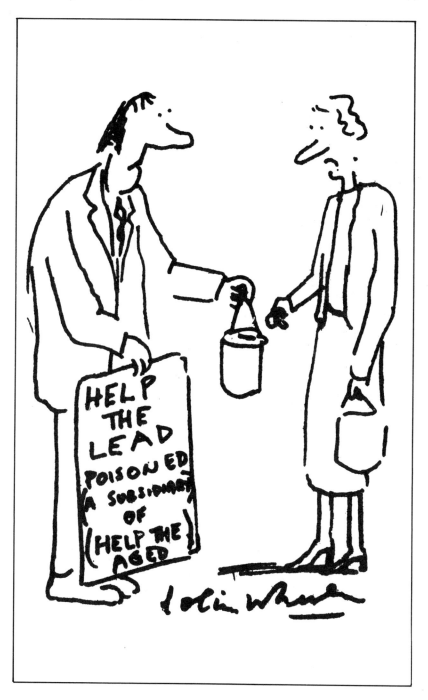

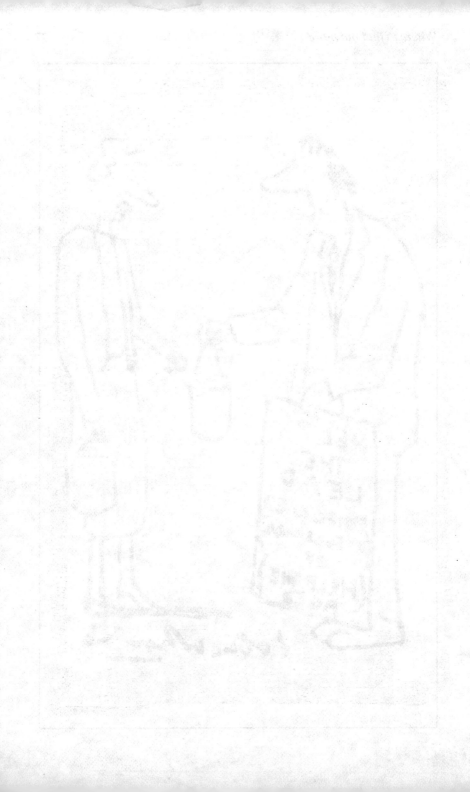

CLEAR

The Campaign for Lead-free Air

The case for a phasing out of lead in petrol is now unanswerable— as this booklet makes clear.

You can help achieve this objective by supporting **CLEAR**, the Campaign for Lead-Free Air.

CLEAR is conducting a nationwide campaign and needs money and also help at local level.

If you would like to help **CLEAR** please write to:

CLEAR
2 Northdown Street
London N1 9BG
Telephone: 01-278 9686

CLEAR

The Campaign for Lead-free Air